Dear Nancy,
May you find joy, solace
and inspiration in our
adventure. Best of health
to you! Andrea Gabbard
12/99

No Mountain Too High

A Triumph Over Breast Cancer

The Story of the Women
of Expedition Inspiration

Andrea Gabbard

Seal Press

Seal Press
3131 Western Avenue, Suite 410
Seattle, WA 98121
sealprss@scn.org

Cover design by Trina Stahl
Cover photographs © by James W. Kay
Text design and composition by Clare Conrad

Library of Congress Cataloging-in-Publication Data
Gabbard, Andrea.
No mountain too high : a triumph over breast cancer /
Andrea Gabbard
1. Breast—Cancer—Patients—United States—Biography.
2. Mountaineering—Argentina. 3. Aconcagua, Mount, (Argentina)
I. Title.
RC280.B8G323   1998   362. 1'9699449'00922—dc21   98-7824
ISBN 1-58005-008-5

Printed in Canada
First printing, July 1998
10 9 8 7 6 5 4 3 2 1

Distributed to the trade by Publishers Group West
In Canada: Publishers Group West Canada, Toronto, Ontario
In the U.K. and Europe: Airlift Book Company, Middlesex, England
In Australia: Banyan Tree Book Distributors, Kent Town, South Australia

This book is dedicated to the women and men of
Expedition Inspiration

Contents

Expedition Inspiration

SUMMIT TEAM

Survivors
Claudia Berryman-Shafer, NV
Vicki Boriack, CA
Laura Evans, ID
Nancy Knoble, CA
Annette Porter, WA
Mary Yeo, ME

Guides
Catie Casson, WA
John Hanron, CA
Heather MacDonald, WA
Jeff Martin, WA
Kurt Wedburg, CA
Peter Whittaker, WA

Support
Dr. Bud Alpert, CA
Paul Delorey, WI
Andrea Gabbard, CA
James Kay, UT
Steve Marts, WA
Jeannie Morris, UT

TREK TEAM

Survivors
Kim O'Meara Anderson, IO
Ashley Sumner-Cox, MT
Claudia Crosetti, CA
Eleanor Davis, PA
Patty Duke, CO
Roberta Fama, CA
Sue Anne Foster, CA
Sara Hildebrand, WI
Nancy Hudson, CA
Nancy Johnson, CA
Andrea Martin, CA

Guides
Larry Luther, UT
Sue Luther, UT
Mike "Ole" Olson, UT
Ned Randolf, WA
Mark "Tuck" Tucker, WA
Jennifer Wedburg, CA
Erika Whittaker, WA

Support
Bill Arnold, IL
Dr. Ron Dom, ID
Roger Evans, ID
Dr. Kathleen Grant, CA
Byron Smith, IL
Saskia Thiadens, CA

Introduction

*The highest art is the art of living an ordinary life
in an extraordinary manner.* —Tibetan saying

Expedition Inspiration's Journey of Hope

The best stories are those about the triumph of the human spirit over adversity. These stories awaken the hero inside each of us, propel us to reach beyond self-imposed limits and inspire us to move mountains—or, climb them.

The story of the women of Expedition Inspiration is one of these stories.

As these stories often go, this one starts with one person, but doesn't end there. This is about seventeen women who took the story and shouted it from the mountaintops. The tale begins with Laura Evans and her battle against breast cancer. It ends in a victory of mind over mountain.

In 1989, at age forty, Laura discovered a lump in her breast during self-examination and went straight to her physician. After examining the lump and ordering a subsequent mammogram, the doctor assured her it was nothing.

"It was what I wanted to hear," said Laura, who had recently returned from a 250-mile hike through Nepal earlier in the year as a member of a trek team that had followed Lou Whittaker's American Kangchenjunga Expedition into base camp. She added, "I felt stronger then than I had ever felt in my life."

Four months later, Laura found a second lump, this one in her armpit. This time the mass wasn't "nothing." It was a dangerous, fast-growing, stage-three cancer that had metastasized to eleven of her lymph nodes. "One day I was scaling peaks and running half-marathons and the next day I learned I had only a fifteen percent chance of surviving the next three to five years," she said. A dedicated fitness buff who ate a low-fat diet and had no history of breast cancer in her family, Laura had always believed that she was as low-risk as they come. Tall, blonde and blessed with an indomitable will, Laura was used to charting her own course in life.

The news not only disrupted Laura's successful career as a freelance fashion and sports apparel designer, it also interrupted a goal that she had been working toward for two years: to climb 19,340-foot Mount Kilimanjaro in Africa with a group of friends on a trip to be led by Peter and Erika Whittaker, owners of Summits Adventure Travel.

Laura was forced to put Kilimanjaro on hold. Determined to beat the odds, Laura and Roger, her husband of twenty years, contacted specialists around the country to find out how she could increase her chances of survival. The answer involved drastic, debilitating treatment, beginning with surgery to remove part of her breast and several lymph nodes. This was followed by what was then an experimental treatment. For seven weeks, Laura was confined to a sterile, six-by-eight-foot hospital room in San Francisco, where she received intensive chemotherapy and bone marrow rescue. The treatment weakened her immune system to a dangerously low level. If she had left that room, she would have died.

Laura endured a life-threatening bout with pneumonia and then contracted lymphedema, a painful and sometimes incapacitating secondary condition that can occur when lymph nodes and vessels are compromised by surgery or radiation. She lost part of her breast and part of her memory. She lost her taste buds, her fingernails, her toenails and every hair on her body.

But she never lost her determination to live and to climb the world's highest mountains. In her hospital room was a window overlooking a tiny park. "Every day," she reflects, "I'd look out that window and tell myself that when I got out I was going to walk through that park." On her first day out of the hospital, in July 1990, she walked the four blocks through that park. Two weeks later, still in San Francisco undergoing radiation treatment, she walked nine miles.

"I didn't really mean to go that far," she said. "I just didn't want to turn around, so I kept going. Once you have a mindset of being physically fit and being outdoors, you never lose it."

She also never lost sight of the lessons she had learned from her illness. "What I really want to tell people is that you don't have to die from cancer," she said. "You can live with a life-threatening illness and go on to achieve unlimited goals."

That September, as planned, Peter led a group of Laura's friends to the summit of Kilimanjaro. Laura was too weak to climb mountains, but she still regarded Kilimanjaro as unfinished business and began working out in earnest. By June 1992, less than two years after her treatment had ceased, she had become strong enough to summit Washington State's Mount Rainier with Peter. There, she realized that she was ready for Kilimanjaro. Peter was leading a trip that fall and encouraged Laura to go.

Four months later, in October 1992, with Peter as her guide, Laura stood atop Uhuru Peak on Mount Kilimanjaro, the highest point on the African continent. Peter tells it this way: "About two hundred feet from the summit, we're all moving slowly, breathing hard, pacing ourselves at high altitude. Laura suddenly stops me and asks, 'Peter, do you think it would be all right if I ran the rest of the way?' Her excitement and joy at having achieved this summit and having regained her health propelled her to the top. It was an incredible display of strength, will and positive spirit."

Laura came down off that peak inspired to climb a mountain for breast cancer research. "I told Peter, I want to climb another mountain, but I want to do it for breast cancer. He was immediately supportive and gave the project its name: Expedition Inspiration."

In August 1993, I first met Laura Evans at a breakfast with our mutual friend, Peter Whittaker. With them was Andrea Martin, also a breast cancer survivor and the founder of the Breast Cancer Fund (BCF) in San Francisco. We were in Reno, Nevada, to attend a trade show for the outdoor industry. I was there in my capacity as senior contributing editor for *Outdoor Retailer* magazine. Laura, Peter and Andrea were there to seek sponsors for their mountaineering expedition.

Because mountaineering expeditions are a fairly regular occurrence these days, there's a lot of competition for sponsors. The fact that all of this planet's major peaks (those over 8,000 meters or 26,000 feet) have been climbed, individually and by teams, nearly every which way but upside down and naked—although that day will probably come—has made securing sponsorships harder than ever.

Climbing big mountains is expensive. Many of the countries in which these mountains are situated, such as China, Nepal, Tibet and Pakistan, have imposed high and stringent fees for climbing permits in order to limit the number of foreigners on their prized and sometimes sacred peaks. Today, you need a unique approach to attract companies to fund an adventurous and risky project. No company wants to underwrite somebody's vacation of a lifetime.

Knowing this, when the three people sitting before me told me of their intent to organize a team of breast cancer survivors to climb the highest mountain in the Western Hemisphere to raise money for breast cancer research, I perked up. Climbing a mountain to raise funds for a worthy cause wasn't a new idea. Earlier that year, a small team of climbers had ascended Mount McKinley in Alaska to raise funds for AIDS research. This Climb for the Cure had raised $250,000, an extraordinary accomplishment for a small, grassroots project. The proposed breast cancer fundraising climb was unique in that it would mark the first time that the actual sufferers of a targeted disease would comprise the team. The expedition also had an ambitious goal of raising $2.3 million—or $100 per foot—by climbing 22,841-foot Mount Aconcagua in Argentina.

And why not climb a mountain? Other fundraising organizations held bike rides, runs, golf tournaments, triathlons—any number of activities to attract attention, participation and donations.

At our breakfast meeting, Andrea Martin explained to me that funds raised would be used to increase awareness of breast cancer and to support cutting-edge projects nationwide that promote breast cancer research, education, policy action, patient support and treatment. Martin had founded the BCF in 1992, after surviving a double mastectomy. Expedition Inspiration would be the project that would launch the BCF into the ranks of viable fundraising entities. Since I was familiar with the various companies in the outdoor industry, Laura, Peter and Andrea asked me for advice on which ones to approach for support. They also asked me to become a member of the Aconcagua summit team. The summit team's goal would be to ascend to the top of the mountain. A separate trek team would hike to the 13,800-foot base camp in support of the summit team.

I had first met Peter while climbing Mount Rainier. At 14,411 feet, Mount Rainier is the highest peak in the Pacific Northwest and is considered to be the most difficult endurance climb in the Lower 48. I believed it. At the time of our meeting in 1993, I had already tried to summit the glaciated peak on four different occasions and hadn't yet succeeded. The first two times, in 1988 and 1989, my physical condition peaked out before the mountain did. On the next two attempts, in 1992 and 1993, bad weather thwarted my dream of standing on the summit. But the outcome of these many attempts had been positive: in 1993, at age 46, I was more physically fit than ever before, and I had gained two new friends in Peter Whittaker and his father, Lou.

As a result of my forays onto the flanks of Mount Rainier, I ended up co-writing Lou Whittaker's life story (*Lou Whittaker, Memoirs of a Mountain Guide*). Lou is a world-famous mountaineer and professional guide and the founder and owner of Rainier Mountaineering, Inc. (RMI), the official guide service in Mount Rainier National Park. Peter was raised with Mount Rainier as his backyard and is a veteran of two Everest expeditions. Peter had become part-owner of RMI and, with his wife, Erika, had also founded an international guide service called Summits Adventure Travel. Summits Adventure Travel would be the outfitting guide service for the Aconcagua climb.

During my work on Lou's autobiography, I relied on Peter's input for a chapter about a tragedy involving a huge icefall that had occurred on Mount Rainier in 1981 in which eleven clients had perished. Peter had been one of the guides on that climb and had never told the full story to anyone outside the official committee that had been formed at the time to investigate the tragedy. By the time he had related the story into my tape recorder, we both were in tears. Like most mountain climbers, Peter has a macho streak and a healthy ego. But he is also a sensitive individual with a soft and caring heart. He takes his responsibility for his clients seriously. As his father often states, "There are lots of good climbers, but very few good guides. A good guide puts his clients' welfare before his own." Because I knew that Peter fit this description, I agreed to be part of the Aconcagua team, although I hadn't yet climbed over 12,300 feet.

"You'll do fine," Peter assured me. And that, for the time being, was that. While little pangs of self-doubt began to ping-pong crazily in my head, I forced myself to concentrate on the continuing discussion of Expedition Inspiration.

While Laura evaluated potential team members and took responsibility for managing the project, Peter would concentrate on the logistics of the climb of Aconcagua as well as practice climbs slated for Mount Rainier in July 1994 and Sun Valley, Idaho, later in October. Together they would seek gear and clothing sponsors in the outdoor industry. Andrea Martin and her year-and-a-half-old Breast Cancer Fund would seek corporate donors, secure a documentary producer and coordinate official fundraising activities by the BCF as well as by team members and other people or organizations who wanted to contribute to the cause.

As it turned out, many individuals and companies stepped up to the plate with offers of money or product. Paul Delorey, president of JanSport, the world's largest manufacturer of daypacks, became the project's greatest supporter. He committed his company to underwriting the entire cost of the expedition. This meant that all money raised by the team would go to research grants rather than to team expenses. In addition, JanSport supplied tents, duffel bags, packs, hats, sweatshirts and T-shirts emblazoned with the Expedition Inspiration logo.

The project had struck a very emotional chord in Paul. When he was ten years old, he had lost his aunt to breast cancer. "After she died, my five young cousins moved in with our family," he says. "At that age, one of the things I understood was that in addition to my five brothers and sisters, I then had five more kids to play with. What I didn't understand at that age was why my cousins would cry themselves to sleep at night."

Paul explained that he had another vested interest in helping to find a cure for breast cancer: "I have a wife, three daughters and about four hundred female employees." Paul would climb Aconcagua with the summit team.

Paul's tentmate would be Dr. Bernard "Bud" Alpert, a leading microvascular and reconstructive surgeon from San Francisco whose mother and mother-in-law both had suffered from breast cancer. Dr. Bud, as he came to be called by the team, had recently climbed Mount Kilimanjaro with his equally active wife, Susan. Both were involved in charitable efforts for breast cancer research.

John Cooley, vice president of Marmot Mountain, Ltd., the supplier of expedition clothing and sleeping bags to the team, would climb Mount Rainier with the summit team. John and his wife, Neide, had recently lost a sister-in-law to breast cancer.

James "Jimmy" Kay, a professional photographer and close friend of Peter, became the official photographer. He would climb with the summit team. His wife, Susie, climbed Rainier with the team, then stayed home to run their photography business while Jimmy spent nearly a month photographing the Aconcagua climb.

Two other doctors would join the trek team: Dr. Kathleen Grant, an oncologist from San Francisco, and Dr. Ron Dorn, a radiation oncologist from the Mountain States Tumor Institute (MSTI) in Boise, Idaho. Kathleen, who happened to be Laura's oncologist, enjoyed trekking with her husband, Tim, a pathologist. The faculty at MSTI had been very active in fundraising with Laura, and Ron, a triathlete, was eager to test his mettle on a mountain climb.

Saskia Thiadens, a nurse and pioneering founder of the National Lymphedema Network in San Francisco, had met Andrea Martin at a BCF fundraiser and had treated Laura for lymphedema. She also had introduced Laura and Andrea. An avid hiker, Saskia became one of the medical professionals on the team.

The summit and trek teams would be led by several professional mountain guides who had been handpicked carefully by Peter and Erika. "We looked for guides who had the heart for an expedition of this type," says Peter. Catie Casson, a wiry, fiery, freckled redhead all of five feet tall and strong enough to carry more than half her weight on her back, had worked for RMI for ten years. She would guide as well as cook for the summit team. Other summit team guides included Kurt Wedburg, a senior guide at RMI with plans to climb Mount Everest three months after Aconcagua, and senior guides John Hanron, Jeff Martin and Heather MacDonald. At age sixteen, Heather had lost her mother to ovarian cancer. Already a veteran of climbs on Mounts Everest and McKinley, Heather, at twenty-five, was extremely motivated to help Expedition Inspiration achieve its goal.

As the team moved closer to the summit, Jeff and Heather would concentrate on lending support to the documentary producer, Jeannie Morris, and her cameraman, Steve Marts. Morris was a former sports broadcaster and seasoned television producer, director and writer. Marts, a veteran mountaineer and videographer, would capture the summit team's journey. To the trek team, Jeannie assigned a separate camera crew, Bill Arnold and Byron Smith.

The trek team would be led by Mark "Tuck" Tucker. A friendly bear of a man, Tuck was another senior guide at RMI and had summited Mount Everest in 1990 as a member of the International Peace Climb led by Peter's uncle, Jim Whittaker. (Jim had become the first American to summit Mount Everest in 1963.)

Tuck would be assisted on Aconcagua by Erika Whittaker and another group of senior RMI guides, including Jennifer Wedburg, Larry and Sue Luther, Mike "Ole" Olson and Ned Randolf.

Mountain guides are accustomed to inspiring their clients. To a person, each guide admitted, "The women of Expedition Inspiration inspired *me.*"

In March 1994, Laura journeyed with Peter and clients of Summits Adventure Travel to climb the twin Mexican volcanoes, Popocatepetl (17,887 feet) and Orizabo (18,701 feet). Afterward, she and Peter talked me into going with them on another trip in May to climb 19,870-foot Huayna Potosí in Bolivia as a training climb for Aconcagua. To my great satisfaction, I reached the summit along with the rest of the group.

Back in our 18,000-foot high camp on Huayna Potosí that night, we were rewarded for our efforts with the sight of a full moon rising in the clear sky above a nearby Andean peak. I was standing beside Laura and noticed that she was crying. I put my arm around her.

She said, "I just thank God that I'm alive to see this."

Four months later, Laura continued her conditioning regime

for Aconcagua by summiting Mount Elbrus (18,498 feet) in Russia. "I felt great the entire time," she said upon her return. "I'm ready for Aconcagua."

At the Reno outdoor trade show, I had introduced Laura, Peter and Andrea Martin to Peg Moline, the editor of *Shape*, the popular women's fitness magazine. Peg had agreed to run an article about Laura and Expedition Inspiration and had slated the story for the Publisher's Page in the March 1994 issue. At the end of the article was a call for applications from breast cancer survivors in top physical condition and with mountaineering experience for the summit team, as well as for survivors in good enough condition to be part of an additional trek team that would undertake a three-day hike to the 13,800-foot base camp on Aconcagua. This article, plus several well-placed ads in other national magazines, referrals from doctors and word of mouth, resulted in nearly two hundred responses. From this outpouring of interest, Laura, Andrea and Peter gradually selected two teams of breast cancer survivors from around the country, six women for the summit team and eleven for the trek team. The team members ranged in age from twenty-one to sixty-one, and included single and married women, single mothers, married mothers and grandmothers. The women were selected on the basis of their experience with breast cancer, their physical ability to trek or climb and their willingness to share their feelings and insights with other team members and with the world in general, through the media.

Learning about each team member's experience with breast cancer was a real education about the nature of breast cancer itself. The types of cancer the women had contracted, the treatments, recovery processes and reconstruction options were as varied as their backgrounds. I learned that the disease truly is indiscriminate. There really is no "model" victim other than that it is more often a woman than a man; for example, in 1993, 182,000 women and 1,000 men were diagnosed with breast cancer.

I learned from BCF statistics that breast cancer has reached almost epidemic proportions, and that in the United States, a woman dies of breast cancer every eleven minutes. In 1994, 1.8 million women in the U.S. had been diagnosed with breast cancer, and a million more did not yet know they had the disease. Breast cancer is the leading cause of death among women ages forty to forty-four and the leading cause of cancer death in women ages fifteen to fifty-four. The death rate from breast cancer has not been reduced in more than fifty years and the incidence of breast cancer among American women continues to rise each year. No one knows what causes breast cancer, how to cure it or what to do to prevent it. The statistics are almost endlessly depressing.

When Peter and Laura asked me to join the team, I was no stranger to cancer. My grandmother had died of stomach cancer in 1970. A close friend had died of metastasized breast cancer in 1985. In 1990, I had cared for my mother as she slowly died of lung cancer after undergoing months of extensive chemotherapy and radiation. In 1991, my father-in-law died of renal cancer. I had witnessed the toll the various treatments take on a person's physical and emotional being, and I was familiar with the effects of cancer on the victim's family and friends. Cancer is the most insidious of diseases, complete with the hopefulness of remission, the dread of recurrence and the fear of death. Families and friends are often infected with an unbearable sense of helplessness and despair, and, finally, guilty relief when the struggle ends.

And yet, among the seventeen breast cancer survivors of the

Expedition Inspiration team, I witnessed an overwhelmingly positive mental attitude to a degree that almost made me wish I were one of them. The experience has given new meaning to the word *team*. We are all in this life experience together. Survival depends on our ability to unite harmoniously to combat the obstacles that appear in our paths.

I also have learned that contracting breast cancer, or any major cancer, often impels an inward journey that rivals, if not exceeds, any imaginable physical venture, including climbing a mountain. For many of the team members, breast cancer sounded a wake-up call, forced them to examine their lives and to put their interior houses in order. Throughout the months that led up to the assault on Aconcagua, there were several gatherings of team members for the purpose of training or to introduce a new team member, to raise funds, to stay in touch and offer support. Often, during these gatherings, we'd form a circle and listen as each woman's inner journey unfolded in heartrending narrative. Each story was heroic and poignant in its own right, and not without a few hearty doses of humor— and hugs. Laughter and affection were an important part of team meetings.

In July 1994, the initial members of Expedition Inspiration gathered for the first time as a team on Mount Rainier for a "shakedown climb" in preparation for Aconcagua. This was when the team members first met each other and the team's unity of spirit first manifested itself. This was where the outward journey began, and established a metaphor for each team member's struggle for life.

During the two years leading up to the Aconcagua climb, Laura was often asked, "Why climb a mountain for breast cancer?"

In response, she would point out that surviving breast cancer and climbing mountains are in many ways analogous. In the book she wrote after the climb, *The Climb of My Life*, she outlined her usual response to the question:

"In climbing a mountain and dealing with breast cancer, you face your deepest fear, the reality of death.

"You have to summon up all your strength physically and emotionally to reach your objective.

"Each is an individual struggle that is more effectively handled with team support.

"In order to survive, it takes one small courageous uphill step at a time.

"In the process, you find out what kind of person you are and what your ultimate values are. You develop a greater sense of self and self-worth."

The story of Expedition Inspiration is the story of seventeen women who survived a life-threatening disease and then put themselves at risk again on one of the world's highest mountains in order to save other lives. Along the way, many personal summits were achieved, many expectations realized and some expectations shattered. For many, the experience of breast cancer and mountain climbing became a spiritual challenge, a metaphysical journey. No one walked away from Aconcagua—or breast cancer—unchanged. In following their lives before and after the climb of Aconcagua, it is my hope that readers will find solace and inspiration, as I have, from the life-affirming spirit, strength and determination exhibited by the women of Expedition Inspiration.

Part One

First Steps

*"I began to realize that I didn't have to hide my cancer
or my pain. I didn't have to go through all this alone.
That was the beauty of being part of the team."*
— Nancy Hudson

Building a Team

On a warm September morning in 1990, in Iowa City, Iowa, thirty-five-year-old Kim O'Meara Anderson gave birth to Evan John, her first and only son. Three months later, she discovered a mass in her left breast. The mass was diagnosed as breast cancer.

Four years later, on July 9, 1994, having survived breast cancer but determined to help find a way to help other women conquer or avoid the disease altogether, Kim flew to Seattle, Washington, to join a group of like-minded women who would comprise the core of Expedition Inspiration. The women's immediate goal was to climb 14,411-foot Mount Rainier in preparation for an expedition the following January that would take them to the highest mountain in the Western Hemisphere, Argentina's 22,841-foot Mount Aconcagua.

In Seattle, Kim quickly realized that she wasn't the only anxious team member. This would be the first time that most of the team members had met. They gathered at Sea-Tac Airport, where Peter Whittaker and one of his senior guides, Mark Tucker, picked them up for the two-and-a-half-hour ride to Ashford, the small mountain community at the entrance to Mount Rainier National Park. By the time the van reached Ashford, the women were well on their way to becoming acquainted. As Patty Duke, a trek team member from Steamboat Springs, Colorado, later said, "I went to Rainier concerned that I wouldn't remember anybody's name and I went home with everybody being my best friend. It was an instant connection—all of us having breast cancer, all of us loving the outdoors and all of us wanting to help other women."

Each time the team met, the women formed a circle and took turns revealing their personal histories and their motivation for joining the team. That most of them did not fit the so-called profile of a cancer victim soon became apparent. Most of the women had no history of any type of cancer in their families. Most had led healthy, active lives. Some were surely "too young." The more the women learned about each other, the more the truth became evident: breast cancer does not heed age or historical health limits.

At the time she joined the team in 1994, thirty-nine-year-old Kim was an artist and teacher in Cedar Rapids, Iowa. She and her husband, Art, had married a year and a half before Evan was born. They both had waited until their thirties to have children. Evan represented the start of their family life.

There had been some breast cancer in Kim's family—a cousin had been diagnosed at age twenty-eight and a great aunt had died of the disease. But Kim's mother and grandmother were free of cancer. "I grew up on a farm in Iowa where pesticide and herbicide use was pretty common," explains Kim, a vegetarian for the past twenty years. "I really think there might be an environmental link to breast cancer." Kim, athletic as well as artistic, with short, blond-highlighted brown hair and a ready smile, had always enjoyed an active lifestyle. In college, she had done a lot of hiking, backpacking and canoeing. She and Art had trekked in Alaska on their honeymoon. Both ran several miles daily and looked forward to camping and hiking with Evan.

Kim heard about Expedition Inspiration on Valentine's Day, 1994. "The first thing I did was think of all the reasons I couldn't do the climb—I have a three-year-old, a marriage to maintain, a full-time job," says Kim. "I called Laura about five times and chickened out and hung up before she answered. Then I realized, 'I can do this if I want to,' and finally called Laura and didn't hang up." Kim was placed on the trek team.

Ashley Sumner-Cox was only eighteen when she was diagnosed in 1991, and twenty-one when she joined the team. During her senior year in high school in Charlottesville, Virginia, she had gone to her family doctor for a breast reduction. "I was a very active kid and I was tired of my breasts getting in the way all the time," says Ashley. "I rode horses, played polo. And I knew that people were always looking at my breasts instead of at me when we were talking. It was really hard and always embarrassing to me."

A routine examination of the breast tissue removed from Ashley revealed cancer. The doctor was astounded that he had found cancer in an eighteen-year-old, and sent tissue samples to six other doctors for confirmation. The unanimous recommendation: a mastectomy. Ashley was stunned and angry, and spent the next year trying to find cancer support groups for young people. "There weren't any," she says. "I'd go to meetings and I'd be the baby. I stuck out. I was this 'Poor girl, poor dear.' All these women were bald, had wigs and stuff. I couldn't deal with it."

After graduating from high school, Ashley moved to Missoula, to attend the University of Montana, and to escape her notoriety as "the youngest breast cancer survivor in Charlottesville." In Missoula, her love of sports quickly translated to hiking, backpacking, climbing and whitewater kayaking. When she heard about Expedition Inspiration, she thought, "What a great way to give back, in honor of all the people who have been so kind to me."

Ashley applied for a position on the trek team, although she had developed aspirations of being a mountain guide herself. "I have a habit of making my expectations low so that I never get disappointed," she says. "I thought I was going to feel alienated because I was the youngest and not going to be able to interact very well with the team. I was afraid that the trek was going to be too hard and I wasn't going to be able to keep up. I had a whole lot of self-doubt. I talked about it to Laura and she reassured me. She also told me not to get any older." Laura understood the promotional value of having such a young breast cancer survivor on the team. Ashley joined the trek team in September 1994, and missed the Mount Rainier shakedown climb. She finally met the team in October, during another training session in Sun Valley, Idaho. Her self-deprecating humor and little-girl demeanor endeared her to the other team members. Ashley became the baby sister of the team.

Two other team members joined after the shakedown climb: Mary Yeo and Nancy Knoble.

Mary Yeo had been diagnosed in the fall of 1989 at age fifty-three. A tall, proud woman graced with a perpetually pleasant expression, Mary was a wife, mother of seven grown children and grandmother of five. There had been some history of breast cancer in her family. "My grandmother had it. My mother didn't. I just never thought I'd get it. I remember hiking with a friend while waiting for the results of my biopsy. I told my friend, 'You know, I don't think I have breast cancer. I feel so good.' No aches or pains, no indications. I had climbed Mount Kenya in Africa that summer and was just breezing happily through my life."

Mary and her husband, Bill, had lived in the small town of Cumberland Center, Maine, for twenty-three years. After teaching for many years, Mary now worked in camping sales at the famous L.L. Bean store in Freeport. Bill was retired from the school system. They had been active all their lives. Bill is an avid fisher and hunter, while Mary has always found time to walk, hike, ski, run or bicycle, and has encouraged her five daughters and two sons to do the same. In fact, her sons had climbed Aconcagua the year before Mary was diagnosed with breast cancer. Mary was fifty-eight when she became a member of the summit team.

Nancy Knoble's experience with breast cancer started in 1983, when she had a biopsy of a tumor on her right breast. The tumor turned out to be benign, but her doctor warned her that it could be a precursor to breast cancer. In 1990, a close friend, Cathie, was diagnosed with breast cancer eight-and-a-half months into her pregnancy. Nancy went through the entire experience with her. "It seemed pretty overwhelming to me," she remembers.

During the following two years, two more friends were diagnosed, one right after the other. "When I was diagnosed in 1993, instead of feeling like, 'Why me?' it was more like, 'Why not me?'" says Nancy. "I was well aware of the statistics by then. It seemed to be happening all around me."

At the time, Nancy was forty-five and vice president of human resources for a communications company in the Bay Area. She lived in Tiburon, an upscale community north of San Francisco. Nancy's husband of nine years, Richard Hinkel, worked as a human resources consultant. Theirs was a second marriage for both, free of the responsibility of children, free to enjoy life to the fullest. They lived an active lifestyle that included running, backpacking and skiing. In addition, they aggressively supported various environmental causes in their community.

Nancy heard about Expedition Inspiration at a Breast Cancer Fund fundraiser in the fall of 1993, when Laura Evans announced the project. She sent in an application, but initially was turned down. "I asked Andrea Martin why I wasn't chosen," says Nancy, who is tall, slender and exceptionally fit. "She asked Laura. Laura told her that my treatment was so recent, she didn't think I'd be strong enough, and that I didn't really have any high altitude climbing experience. Richard and I had climbed Mount Rainier in 1992 and had done lots of backpacking in the Sierras, so I felt qualified. Laura also said there were already so many women from the Bay Area on the team; she wanted the team to be more national in scope."

Laura and Andrea also wanted the team to have more ethnic diversity, and were actively seeking women of color for the team. Breast cancer is particularly deadly among minorities who are also underprivileged. Many researchers attribute this fact more to lack of information and unavailability of screening than to genetic predisposition. A Bay Area African-American woman was being considered at the time. Meanwhile, Nancy Knoble continued to train and even journeyed to Russia in the fall of 1994 to climb 18,498-foot Mount Elbrus with Laura on a trip led by Summits Adventure Travel. When the African-American candidate decided that her busy schedule would not allow her to participate, Laura finally relented and accepted Nancy on the summit team.

"I had never given up hope," says Nancy. "I knew I would be a part of the expedition in one way or another, even if it meant helping other people train or raising funds. I knew I was meant to be part of it."

Claudia Crosetti and Nancy Johnson of Ukiah, California, were the first team members to be selected by Laura. Claudia's oncologist, Dr. Kathleen Grant, also happened to be Laura Evans's oncologist and informed Claudia of the expedition in August 1993. "You're one of my more athletic patients," said Dr. Grant, "so I thought you'd be interested."

Claudia had been diagnosed two years before, at age thirty-eight, while working as an administrative assistant at the local junior college. During her recuperation, she sought a support group, but, as she explains, "There weren't many breast cancer patients, just cancer patients in general. I think I would have benefited more if we'd had the commonality of the body image and treatment issues."

Eventually, Claudia met Nancy Johnson, who had been diagnosed in 1990. "We both were into physical activity, such as playing tennis, running, race walking, swimming," Claudia says. "So we thought, why don't we do that together? We can talk about our cancer experience while we're doing physical things. We became our own support group, and later started a breast cancer support group in Ukiah."

In 1990, Nancy Johnson had recently moved into a new house in Ukiah with her partner of four years, Janet. Nancy, an energy consultant, led an active, healthy lifestyle, but, like Kim, had grown up on a farm in the Midwest. "In Illinois, when I was twelve, I worked in the corn fields with other kids my age," says Nancy. "We were sprayed with pesticides over a period of three summers. It was common practice, then. I often wonder how many of the other girls on my detasseling crew ended up with some kind of cancer. There is a high incidence of cancer in my hometown. Much of it has been traced to pesticide exposure."

When Claudia and Nancy applied for the team, they were afraid that Laura wouldn't choose two people from the same town. "Claudia said, 'I think we should both go for it. If I get picked, great. If you get picked, you say, 'No, I can't go unless Claudia goes.' Or, 'No, I've got to let my friend Claudia go because she applied first,'" Nancy explains, smiling. "That was our deal."

Laura interviewed both Claudia and Nancy in San Francisco at the Komen Foundation's annual Race for the Cure in September 1993. "We showed her photos from the walk-a-thon we had organized in Ukiah," says Nancy. "We had raised five thousand dollars for our local breast cancer organization. Laura was looking for people who had a passion for fundraising and she could tell we were real open about talking about our breast cancer experiences. Luckily, she chose both of us for the trek team."

Nancy and Claudia trained together for Rainier and Aconcagua and became close friends. They complemented each other. Claudia is tall and dark-haired; Nancy is average height with blond hair. Claudia's humor is quick and irreverent; Nancy's is more subtle. "We were out there together in Ukiah on 103-degree days, carrying our packs up and down the local hills, encouraging each other," says Nancy.

"I'd never done any backpacking, so I was able to bounce a lot of stuff off Nancy," says Claudia. "I don't know what it would have been like if only one of us had been chosen."

"*You* would've had a good time," Nancy says, in their typical shared banter.

The team could tell by the ever-present smile on Claudia Berryman-Shafer's face that she always had a good time—or, in the least, she always focused on the positive aspects of a situation. Claudia B-S, as the team called her—or Claudia "No B-S" for her straightforward manner—had been diagnosed in the winter of 1993, at age forty-four. Thirty years earlier, her mother had undergone a mastectomy for breast cancer. "We never talked about it," recalls Claudia. "My brothers and I knew she had it, but we didn't go around talking about it. I never even saw her scar. She was in the hospital for nine days, then came home and went back to work."

Claudia B-S has her mother's determination. She was out of the hospital two days after her mastectomy and four days later ran a ten-miler, as she says, "with those stupid drains still in me. I just taped them to my side so that I could run. From the beginning, I had decided that cancer wasn't going to stop me."

Claudia B-S and her husband, Jim, live and teach in Fernley, Nevada, and are ultramarathoners. They train by running every day, ten miles before school and five miles after, and are regular participants in the Leadville Trail 100, a one-hundred-mile foot-race in Colorado that peaks at 12,600 feet elevation. They also enjoy skiing, mountain biking and backpacking, and have worked as wilderness rangers in the Sierra Nevada Mountains during summers. In 1983, together they climbed Alaska's 20,340-foot

Mount McKinley. Claudia also climbed McKinley in 1982, before meeting Jim.

A friend told Claudia B-S about Expedition Inspiration and urged her to submit an application. At the time, Claudia was still undergoing chemotherapy. "Laura called and asked me a few questions about being strong enough since I was still in chemo," says Claudia. "I explained the activities I was doing, including marathons, and Laura said that Peter would call me."

He didn't. As soon as Peter read Claudia's McKinley credentials, he stated, "She's in." Claudia B-S joined the summit team in late May 1994, at age forty-five, strong in both spirit and body.

Sue Anne Foster's credentials included a climb of Africa's 19,340-foot Mount Kilimanjaro. "I didn't mention that I had done it twenty-two years earlier while serving in the Peace Corps," she laughs. "After a mastectomy, eight months of chemo, six weeks of radiation and much inactivity, the climb was the first exciting and positive thing I had encountered related to cancer. I imagined how perfect this would be to help me focus on getting back into shape and reclaiming my body."

Sue Anne had been diagnosed in 1992, when she was forty-seven. Sue Anne lived in Carmichael, a suburb of Sacramento, California, with her husband, Gary, her daughters Mignon, age eleven, and Genevieve, eight, and a menagerie that included two cats, two dogs and a family of African Gray Parrots, the matriarch of which Sue Anne had brought home from Africa after her Peace Corps stint. With a Ph.D. in education and a Master's Degree in art, specializing in art therapy, Sue Anne taught creativity at the local junior college and also worked as an art therapist.

Sue Anne lobbied hard to become a team member. Along

with her resume—"Who would have thought that having breast cancer would be an asset on a resume!" she says—she sent pictures of herself superimposed onto the team's promotional poster and also offered to be the team masseuse. "I think that cinched it," she says, with typical dry humor. Five weeks before the Rainier shakedown climb, Laura called Sue Anne to tell her she had been accepted on the trek team. With her passionate dedication to natural health, vegetarianism and social causes, Sue Anne was affectionately dubbed the team's "hippie."

Patty Duke's sons, Ben and Ryan, were fifteen and ten when Patty was diagnosed in October 1992. Patty, forty-three, was a former model—who still looked like one—and now clothing designer headquartered in Steamboat Springs, Colorado. She and her husband, Peter, were avid skiers and hikers.

"The news really devastated my family," says Patty. "I was the youngest of five children. It seemed backwards. My brothers and sisters wondered, 'Why Patty, the youngest?'" Patty's mother was seventy-nine, in robust health. Patty's father had died only a few years before. During her recovery, she informed her husband that they must simplify their lives: "No more sweaters, no more hats. We're doing socks only," Patty told him. They named their sock company Smart Wool for the product's inherent no-itch properties.

In 1994, a friend told Patty about Expedition Inspiration. Patty sent away for information, thinking she would donate some wool socks to the climbers. "When I got the application, I realized it was asking for breast cancer survivors to be on the team, so I filled it out right away." Knowing her physical limitations, Patty applied for the trek team. She had become afflicted with rheumatoid arthritis as a result of her cancer treatment.

"I really didn't think Laura would choose me, but I sent in the application anyway," says Patty. "It was then that I also decided that regardless of the outcome, it was time to do the things I had often thought of doing, but hadn't. I started a breast cancer support group in Steamboat and organized a river walk for breast cancer to be added to the Steamboat Marathon in June. When I became lost or confused in my attempts to organize these things, I'd call Laura and ask for help. She had started a support group in Sun Valley and offered good advice. During one of our conversations, she told me I had made the team. Peter and the boys had to peel me off the ceiling!"

Patty's husband was skeptical about her chances of making the trek to Aconcagua's base camp because of the rheumatoid arthritis. Patty says, "He would watch me hobble around, come down the stairs backwards in the morning because my ankles were so stiff, and he'd say, 'You'll never make it.' That just gave me more incentive."

Sara Hildebrand's husband, Fritz, supported Sara's decision to apply for the team. Sara had been jolted by her diagnosis of breast cancer in 1993, at age sixty. "Fritz is a marathoner, so we eat a very healthy diet," she explains. "Exercise is part of our lifestyle. I had no cancer in my family, I was in perfectly good health. I had answered, 'No,' to every question on the pre-surgery questionnaire except the one that asked, 'What did you do aerobically in your twenties?' I had to write, 'Nothing,' because the word aerobics wasn't around forty years ago. We had four children up in a third-floor apartment, while Fritz was in medical school and completing his residency. We didn't know anything. We were all smoking, for one thing. I smoked until I was thirty, when I went for a physical and the doctor told me,

'You're in great shape, but don't smoke anymore. We're learning now that smoking isn't good for you.' I walked out of his office and never smoked another cigarette. I stayed active raising my children and playing tennis, but I didn't do anything aerobic until I was fifty, when I started running four miles a few times a week along Lake Winnebago, where we live. So where did the breast cancer come from?"

Sara had read about Expedition Inspiration in *The Milwaukee Sentinel* one morning in February 1994, five months after her mastectomy. "I realized that JanSport, the sponsoring company, was right in my backyard! The headquarters are in Appleton, next door to Neenah. I called for an application right away.

"There are some things in life you know you shouldn't do or you're not sure you even want to do," Sara adds. "With this, I really didn't hesitate. I was delighted to be able to put my energy into something positive. I filled out that application and had it in the mail the same day. Fritz came home that night and I showed him a copy. He said, 'You're in great shape. There's nothing wrong with you. You can do that.' Then I called my oncologist. He said, 'Go for it, you're all right.' I told him, 'I know it!'" In addition to running several times a week, Sara had trekked in Nepal in 1992 and climbed 19,340-foot Mount Kilimanjaro with Fritz in 1990. "I knew I could get to fourteen thousand feet on Aconcagua," Sara says. "I applied for the trek team. I told Laura, 'It's good for people to know that you don't have to be thirty to do everything.'" A petite and stylish mother of four and grandmother of two, Sara became the oldest—and spunkiest—team member at age sixty-one.

Eleanor Davis of Berwyn, Pennsylvania was forty in 1979 when she discovered a lump in her breast. Then, breast cancer was still very much "in the closet"; no one talked about it and mammograms were not routinely prescribed nor widely available. After a mastectomy and a year of chemotherapy, doctors recommended a prophylactic mastectomy of her remaining breast. "I decided to go ahead and do it," she says. "I really believe that's why I'm alive today—because I don't have any breast tissue left."

At the time, Eleanor's husband, Hal, was building a successful real estate development business. They had three young children: Peter, age twelve, Martha, fifteen, and Chris, sixteen. After her surgeries and treatment, Eleanor finished the nursing degree that she had begun before her diagnosis. She immersed herself in raising her children, nursing and working as a volunteer for the American Cancer Society, to help other women.

Eleanor heard about Expedition Inspiration from a friend, Renata Whitaker, who was an ardent supporter of the project. At first, Eleanor felt hesitant to dredge up the past. "I was comfortable helping other people," she says. "I had been doing hospice work and bereavement counseling as well, but I wasn't sure I wanted to relive my own experience. I sent for the application anyway, and after reading it, I realized that there would be a commonality, that we would speak of our experiences with no explaining needed. I knew I could speak about what chemo felt like, about the feelings of worry and fear of death, and the vulnerability that all of us experience. I knew there would be trust. So I applied for the trek team." At fifty-five, Eleanor was physically fit with a lively sense of humor. She enjoyed golfing, skiing and hiking, and had also climbed Kilimanjaro in 1992 with Hal and their family.

The only climbing Andrea Martin had done before Expedition Inspiration was the stairs to her office. Her petite physical stature did not diminish her zeal for the breast cancer cause. At her first meeting with Laura and Peter at the Airport Hilton in San Francisco, she was impressed and intrigued by the project outlined before her. She recalls, "They're talking to me about climbing this huge mountain to raise money for breast cancer research and I'm a person who has never even been camping. The fundraiser in me said, Let's raise a hundred dollars a foot and call it 'The 23,000-foot Assault on Breast Cancer.' I believed if I could help raise nineteen million for Dianne Feinstein's campaign in a year, I could certainly raise over two million dollars for breast cancer in two years." The project would eventually provide an eye-opening contrast between people's willingness to donate money to health-related causes versus political ones.

Andrea Martin had been diagnosed in January 1989 with a tumor in her breast the size of a golfball. After her mastectomy, she had joined Dianne Feinstein's 1990 gubernatorial campaign and succeeded in raising millions of dollars, only to watch Feinstein lose the election by three percentage points. In 1991, just as Feinstein was beginning her bid for the U.S. Senate, Andrea found a lump in her remaining breast. She chose to have that breast removed, also.

The experience with breast cancer "shook me to my foundation," Andrea acknowledges. At the time of her first mastectomy, she was forty-two, she had recently married her second husband, Richard, and she was raising a six-year-old daughter, Mather. "I've had incredible, intimate moments with my husband, daughter and friends that probably wouldn't have happened had I not had such a close brush with death," she adds. "Cancer profoundly changed me forever."

Andrea's experience with cancer also gave her the resolve to follow a new path that led toward her present career as founder and director of the Breast Cancer Fund in San Francisco. At the time of the Rainier shakedown, Andrea's busy schedule had not allowed her time to train, and she wisely elected to forego the climb.

Vicki Boriack rarely passed up an opportunity to climb or simply to get outdoors. A single mother with two teenagers— Katy, fourteen, and Jonathan, twelve—Vicki had been diagnosed in October 1993. For the past six years, she had been separated from her husband, Rod, who lived in Chicago. Vicki and her children lived in Santa Cruz, California, where Vicki worked for MontBell, a company that manufactured outdoor gear and clothing.

Vicki was an active outdoorsperson, involved in backpacking, hiking and river rafting. With a light sprinkling of freckles and bouncy, shoulder-length brown hair, she looked much younger than her thirty-nine years. Although she led a healthy lifestyle, she did have a history of cancer in her family, including her father, who had survived prostate cancer five years before. An aunt had also died of breast cancer in 1993. "The funny thing was," says Vicki, "I'd stand in front of the mirror and say to myself, 'I don't *look* as if I have cancer.'"

A friend told her about Expedition Inspiration. At the time, Vicki was still undergoing chemotherapy and worried that she wouldn't regain her strength in time for Aconcagua. "I would be climbing only seven months after ending chemo," she says. "I discussed it with Laura and we agreed. If by August my body wasn't responding to training, I would step off the team and let someone else go." Although Vicki's extensive outdoor experience qualified her for the summit team, at the time of the Mount Rainier shakedown climb, she had just finished chemotherapy six weeks earlier, and decided to climb only part way with the team.

∾

Nancy Hudson of Ross, California also was a young, single mother when she was diagnosed in 1989. At age thirty-seven, Nancy had recently separated from her husband. She worked as an art consultant, raised funds for local charities and stayed busy raising her two sons—Nick, five, and David, eight.

Nancy was diagnosed right after helping a close friend through her ordeal with breast cancer. The illness, she said, taught her to be nicer to herself. "I was used to doing volunteer work, doing a lot for others, a lot of fundraising for Marin County General Hospital," she states. "I realized that this can become a way of avoiding dealing with yourself, always doing for others and shoving your way through life. Also, it became clear to me just how much superficiality exists in this so-called upper class community. I really started to concentrate on eliminating the superficial stuff and looking harder at giving to myself."

One of her gifts to herself was the commitment to Expedition Inspiration. When she was accepted for the trek team, Nancy was forty-two and fully recovered from breast cancer. A tall, athletic skier and tennis player and a talented fundraiser, Nancy was very motivated to be part of the team.

Roberta Fama of San Mateo, California, was not motivated. "I was always the last person chosen in high school to be on a team," she explains. "My idea of a workout was to dance the night away. I agreed to join the trek team because I was a board member of the Breast Cancer Fund and Andrea Martin asked me to go."

Roberta, now thirty-five and working at Merrill Lynch, had been diagnosed eight years earlier, right after her wedding. "It was all so removed from where my life was going," she says. "I was newly married. We were planning to start a family. Dominic and I had dated for seven years and decided to get married because we wanted to have children. We had their names picked, everything was set. We had our whole lives planned out and this wasn't part of the plan."

Roberta's ordeal with breast cancer stretched over nearly ten years. Two-and-a-half years after her first diagnosis, she had a recurrence in her spine that required more surgery and treatment. In 1992, doctors discovered a large cyst on her ovary and, because of her history, recommended a hysterectomy, thus ending Roberta and Dominic's plans to have children. Roberta's marriage eventually disintegrated under the strain of her illnesses, and she became a team member as a newly-single woman. Gentle, slim and soft-spoken, Roberta's resolve to help other women survive breast cancer was as solid as the mountain she claimed she didn't want to climb.

Annette Porter also was a single career woman when she was diagnosed in February 1991. She was thirty-two and on a fast-track career in human resources management with a large consulting firm in Seattle. Her experience with breast cancer took her to a whole new level of awareness, she acknowledges. "It brought up all sorts of issues for me, including the whole issue of being bald—from chemotherapy—which is connected to your sense of self-worth and femininity and what you look like. All that ended up being tied together. I chose to process that through photography." Since then, as a way to celebrate, Annette has been photographing women—including herself—going through chemotherapy. "We're saying, 'It doesn't have to be with a hat and a wig and a scarf. It can be bald. It can be okay.'"

Annette was the only summit team member with no climbing experience. Tall and energetic, she worked out in a gym and enjoyed in-line skating and cycling, but had not set foot on a mountain trail. She happened to be in New York City on business in January 1994, during an Expedition Inspiration press conference at the Explorer's Club. She attended and was "completely impassioned," she remembers. "I realized the climb was about the celebration of life."

Introducing herself to Peter, Annette told him she had no climbing experience but was willing to do whatever it would take to be a team member. He asked, "Can you growl?"

Although surprised, Annette threw back her mane of light brown hair and growled. Peter said, "Do you want to climb to the summit?"

"Yes!" Annette exclaimed.

"Then you'll do it," he said.

Peter's criteria was a little different from Laura's. In Annette, Peter said he saw "a together person. I knew she would listen to instruction. She looked reasonably active and fit and had the right mindset."

Because of Annette's lack of experience in the mountains, Laura wanted to place her on the trek team. Peter said, "Let's give her a chance. If she summits Rainier during the shakedown climb, that will be the real test."

The shakedown climb proved to be much more than a test—not only for Annette, but for Laura Evans and her entire team of survivors.

Mountain of Triumph

AT 14,411 FEET, MOUNT RAINIER is the largest volcano in the Cascade Range and the largest mountain on the continent in terms of bulk of rock masses, extent of base and number of glaciers. Rainier's twenty-six glaciers form the largest glacial system radiating from a single peak in the world. The mountain towers above the surrounding landscape and can often been seen from as far away as Seattle, Tacoma and Yakima. Locals refer to Mount Rainier as, simply, "the mountain." On a clear day, Seattle residents say, "The mountain is out" to describe the sight of the white, rounded summit dome that seems to hang suspended in the sky.

Mount Rainier has been described by geologists as "an Arctic island in a temperate sea." Climatic zones range from humid rain forests to conditions similar to the Arctic Circle, within a few miles of each other.

Not surprisingly, Mount Rainier generates its own weather. It sits in the path of marine air currents from the Pacific Ocean, which regularly deposit a thick blanket of snow on the upper slopes and generous rainfall in the forests surrounding the mountain during any month of the year. To be able to spend a week on the mountain without experiencing a change in the weather is highly unusual. Glorious sunshine can give way to a raging blizzard within a matter of hours. Storms lay siege to the mountain for days, then abruptly clear away. While lenticular clouds rotate on the summit cap, generating winds in excess of sixty miles per hour, a climber can bask in eighty-degree heat at 10,000-foot Camp Muir. Lou Whittaker, chief guide on the mountain since 1968, attributes this vagary to the mountain "showing off."

In Ashford, the mountain is not visible, a blessing in disguise to some of the more nervous Expedition Inspiration team members. It wasn't until the team van started driving up the winding road through Mount Rainier National Park that the mountain revealed itself, but only in glimpses. Here and there, at a bend in the road, the vast, glaciated peak would suddenly loom through a break in the dense forest. At each view, the mountain seemed to grow bigger. Upon reaching the settlement called Paradise, at the base of the mountain, the landscape opened to reveal the massive, glaciated flanks and crevasse-scarred upper reaches that have enticed climbers and adventurers since the mountain was first climbed in 1852.

To the team members of Expedition Inspiration, Mount Rainier was both inviting and intimidating. The fact that Laura and Peter had termed the exercise a "shakedown climb" added to the performance anxiety that now pervaded most of the group. The first day on the mountain would be spent at "school," learning mountaineering technique. Afterward, we would return to the Nisqually Lodge in Ashford for one more night of rest in a comfortable bed. The following day, we would start climbing the mountain.

When the team van first arrived at the Nisqually Lodge, Laura was standing outside, anticipating our arrival. "Is that Laura?" asked one of the team members. "I can hardly wait to meet her; we've only talked on the phone." Laura beamed as her carefully chosen teammates disembarked and surrounded her, talking, laughing and hugging.

Laura encouraged everyone to check in, freshen up and then meet in the lobby. She had lots of information and bags full of team gear from the various sponsors to disperse.

Roberta Fama and I roomed together. We had already met on a few outings with other California team members. Roberta was excited about meeting the rest of the team, but extremely worried about how she would measure up.

"I was looking forward to meeting Vicki Boriack, another woman with performance anxiety," Roberta told me. "I knew she had just finished chemo and lived not far from me, in Santa Cruz. I was sort of disappointed to find out that she was a mountain woman."

During the van ride from the airport, Roberta confessed that the team's initial reaction to her breast cancer story had been somewhat disconcerting. "I felt them pull away and I thought, 'My God, I'm going to be all alone on this climb,' but eventually they began to warm up and it was fine. It's the initial horror of recurrence—nobody wants to think about that."

A couple of weeks before the Rainier climb, Roberta had called me, concerned that she wouldn't be able to carry a backpack on the mountain. She had filled a little daypack with about twenty pounds of cat litter and worked out with that on her back. Then she heard from another team member that they expected to carry at least forty pounds in their packs during the trek. Roberta panicked. First she called Laura, who, Roberta says, became exasperated.

"Nobody told me you had a bad back," Laura said.

"I don't have a bad back," Roberta responded, "but my muscles have atrophied since my surgery. I need more time."

"This is a problem. We can't pay for a guide to carry your stuff," said Laura.

Roberta replied, "All I can tell you is that I will do my best."

When Roberta called me, she was ready to quit the team. I told her that she'd be given a different type of pack to carry on Rainier and Aconcagua, a full-framed pack with a wide hip belt that was built to carry heavier weight. As soon as we arrived in Ashford, Laura gave her a brand-new JanSport external frame pack. That first night, Roberta filled the pack, tried it on and smiled in relief.

Vicki roomed with Claudia B-S in Ashford. After checking in, she came to our room. "Guess what, my roommate is still in chemotherapy." Vicki looked downcast. "She's strong, she's a marathoner and she's climbed McKinley. And look at me, I finished chemo about six weeks ago and I'm not even going to try to climb to the summit of Rainier."

Vicki wore her heart and her insecurities on her sleeve. She processed her feelings aloud, set limits for herself and often exceeded them, but not without inner struggle. Her honesty and openness were admirable. At times, the anxiety or concern she expressed was shared by others on the team who had chosen instead to keep their feelings to themselves.

Vicki almost had removed herself from the team before the

Rainier shakedown climb. "I finished chemo in June and then started thinking, 'I shouldn't do this. I've got to recover first.' I called Laura right before Rainier and told her of my fears. I wasn't trying to get out of Aconcagua, but she extrapolated that from our conversation. Within a ten-minute conversation, I was off the trip and off the team. It was summer, the kids were gone to their dad's and I cried that whole night and the next. Three days later, I realized I wanted to feel this sort of conviction for everything in my life. I called Laura back. She apologized for jumping to conclusions and agreed that I would go to Rainier, but only climb part-way."

In time, all the women were able to share the anxiety they felt at the initial team gathering. Eleanor told me that she had been "scared to death" when she arrived in Seattle. "I had never been there, I didn't know anyone. I was in pretty good shape but not the kind of shape you're in when you go on a climb. I had read all the team members' bios—Claudia Crosetti and her speed walking, Claudia B-S and her climbing McKinley—and I had to keep telling myself, 'It doesn't make any difference. You're here. It will be okay.' Once we got together, we started opening up and bonding, and I relaxed."

Kim knew she was fit, but wondered, was she fit enough? "I was afraid I wouldn't cut it," she admits. "All the letters from Laura, telling us to train, train, train, be tough, tough, tough, and this is the shakedown climb. I've always been athletic and I've been competitive, but as I get older, I realize that competition is not really all it's cracked up to be. As a runner, you compete more with personal best, which I think is a healthier form of competition.

"I had this idea that the other team members would be Amazon-type women," Kim adds. "Sara Hildebrand—her name conjured up a Nordic woman in braids. Once I met her, I realized,

'She's normal, like me,' and I felt better. We were all normal women, all in the same boat."

Being in the same "boat"—or van, tent or motel room—prompted many of the women to start experiencing hot flashes together, a phenomenon that we observed whenever the team got together. Many of the women had been plunged into early menopause as a result of their cancer treatment. As soon as one would have a hot flash, it would set off another, and so on. The windows would fly open, and off would come jackets and sweatshirts. Claudia B-S's face would flush beet red, a brilliant complement to her bright grin.

That first day in Ashford, after she handed out team gear and clothing, Laura announced that there would be a team dinner that night at which everyone would have a chance to formally introduce herself to the group. Seated together at a long table with the guides and support team members, each survivor took her turn, briefly telling the story of her illness and the reason she had applied for the team.

Nancy Hudson told me later that she was initially depressed at the Nisqually gathering. "My husband and I had separated and my self-esteem was at an all-time low. I thought, 'Oh God, I have to get up and go through the drill, the 'I-am-Nancy-Hudson-and-I-live-in-Ross-and-I-have-two-boys-and-I-like-to-play-tennis-and-ski' routine. Then, listening to everyone who went before me, I suddenly realized this is not what they're talking about at all. These women are talking about their feelings. That was a new experience for me, touching base with other women. I'd never been in a support group. I come from a family of male doctors. They think all that emotional stuff is meaningless. You have your surgery, then shut up and get on with your life. With the team, I began to realize that I didn't have to hide my cancer or my pain. I didn't have to go through all this alone. That was the beauty of being part of the team."

Laura's analogy of surviving breast cancer and climbing a mountain as "an individual struggle that is more effectively handled with team support" found a roomful of proponents that evening.

The following day, July 10, was the team's first day on Mount Rainier. Peter and the RMI guides conducted climbing school, which turned out to be fun as well as instructive. Sue Anne recalls, "I hadn't hiked since I got married. When they handed me an ice ax and crampons, I asked, 'What are these?' I honestly didn't know what gaiters were. I'm sure the look on my face was not that of a person ready to charge up a mountain."

Peter wasn't concerned. He and the RMI guides were used to teaching novices. "They marched us up the mountain," says Sue Anne. "We trained. They had us slide down a hill and do self-arrest with the ice ax. We self-arrested over and over again, head first, back first, upside down and backwards. There was never a thought that you couldn't do it, because you *had* to do it."

Peter was elated to have the team on his turf. At one point, when the women were spread out on a slope and practicing technique, he suddenly executed a perfect backflip in the snow. "How do you like my playground?" he exclaimed.

Training took the edge off the team members' anxiety. With the guides' patient instruction, we learned to execute a self-arrest, by digging our ice ax and boots into the snow to stop a fall. We learned to yell "Falling!" if we fell or saw someone else fall. We practiced walking in crampons, which are spiked metal frames that strapped onto our boots and bit into the snow and ice for greater traction. We roped together in teams of five and six and practiced rope travel uphill and down, and learned rope "courtesy" to avoid jerking the person ahead or behind off her feet.

The guides also taught us two other valuable techniques, pressure breathing and the rest-step, to maximize the body's energy output. Pressure breathing involves a loud exhalation of breath to empty your lungs and make room for more air when you inhale. To do the rest-step, as soon as you swing your front leg forward and put it down with no weight on it, you straighten the back leg and lock the knee so that the bones are in vertical alignment. By resting your weight on that rear leg, you transfer your body weight off your muscles and onto your skeletal structure. The second or two involved in making this shift from muscle to bone support gives your leg muscles a rest. Used together, pressure breathing and rest-stepping create quite an efficient "machine" for climbing. As several team members would discover on Aconcagua, in high altitude where the atmospheric pressure is lower and oxygen deprivation is a normal condition, a climber often needs to take several pressure breaths between each step.

During this first day on Rainier, the mountain showered us with clear, warm and sunny weather, topped off by a welcome light breeze in the afternoon. We basked in perfect climbing weather—now, if only it would hold.

At day's end, a team of suntanned faces with proud grins returned to the RMI Guide Hut at Paradise. There, Peter treated us to a preview of Aconcagua with slides he had taken on a previous trip. After looking at several images of the massive red chunk of South American rock and the arid landscape that blanketed its base, the team members became uncharacteristically silent.

As we walked out of the Guide Hut toward the restaurant at the Paradise Inn, some of the women commented on how "barren and ugly" Aconcagua looked, such a contrast after having spent a day in the pristine snow of Rainier. One of us said, "It looks like a big pile of rocks."

Another remarked, "I thought there would be more snow."

"I'm glad I'm only going to 14,000 feet," said another.

One team member brought us back to the present with an important observation: "Since we're climbing tomorrow and exerting so much energy, we could indulge in dessert tonight. Anyone want to share one with me?"

That night, the team took up two long tables in the Paradise Inn dining room and attracted the attention of several other diners. Many of them asked about the T-shirts emblazoned with the Breast Cancer Fund, Expedition Inspiration, and Aconcagua.

When informed of the team's intent to climb the highest mountain in the Western Hemisphere to raise funds for breast cancer research, one diner confided that his sister had recently found out that she had breast cancer. Could we send her some information? Laura took his name and address and promised to send a press packet. This became a common occurrence whenever the team was out in public. We encountered so many people whose lives were touched in one way or another by breast cancer—a wife, a mother, a sister, a grandmother, a daughter, a friend, the individual herself. The fact that the disease was nearly of epidemic proportion was continually reinforced.

That night, the Nisqually Inn was full of happy, tired climbers dreaming of white slopes and sunshine. Initial impressions of Aconcagua had dissipated over dessert and reassuring remarks from Peter, "Don't worry about Aconcagua," he grinned. "First you have to climb Rainier."

The following day, dawn lit a cloudless sky as we assembled in front of the lodge with our gear. "A summit day," Peter announced. "Let's hope we have a couple more of these."

The plan was for the summit team to carry its gear from Paradise at 5,420 feet to Camp Muir base camp at 10,000 feet, set up tents and make an attempt on the summit from there. The trek team would establish its camp at 6,000 feet on the Nisqually Glacier, then climb to Camp Muir to meet the summit team as it descended from the top.

This game plan approximated the one to be used on Aconcagua. The summit team would hike in first, with the goal of going all the way to the 22,841-foot summit. The trek team would follow five days later and hike to Aconcagua base camp at 13,800 feet. If all went as planned, the trek team would arrive in base camp a day or two before the summit team attempted to reach the top of the mountain. Division of the team not only allowed more breast cancer survivors of varying physical stamina to participate in the expedition, it also lessened the logistical challenge of organizing and transporting forty-two climbers, with all their gear and food, from airport to hotel to trailhead and up the mountain.

At the time of the Mount Rainier shakedown climb, the trek team, which was led by Mark "Tuck" Tucker and Erika Whittaker, included breast cancer survivors Roberta Fama, Nancy Hudson, Nancy Johnson, Claudia Crosetti, Eleanor Davis, Sara Hildebrand, Patty Duke, Kim O'Meara Anderson and Sue Anne Foster. Ashley Sumner-Cox would join the team in the fall. Climbing in support of the trek team were Devra Davis, an epidemiologist from Washington, D.C., and Laura's husband, Roger Evans, a real estate broker.

Roger epitomized the supportive spouse. He remained at Laura's side throughout her cancer ordeal and was her most devoted supporter. He often said in reference to his determined wife, "Cancer picked the wrong person." Roger would also travel to Aconcagua with the trek team.

On the shakedown climb, the only breast cancer survivors on

the summit team led by Peter Whittaker were Laura, Claudia Berryman-Shafer, Annette Porter and Vicki Boriack. Mary Yeo and Nancy Knoble would be added to the team about three months later. Climbing in support were Paul Delorey of JanSport, Dr. Bud Alpert, John Cooley of Marmot Mountain, Ltd., photographers Jimmy and Susie Kay, nurse Saskia Thiadens and myself.

Those of us who had been chosen early for the team had been able to train for the shakedown climb several months in advance. Others, such as Claudia B-S, Sue Anne, Patty and Eleanor, had only a month or two to prepare. To their regular fitness regimes they added the routine of carrying a loaded backpack up and down hills, which is one of the best ways to train for a climb.

As the team van drove into Paradise, we were greeted by a small group of newspaper reporters and local TV newscasters, as well as by various well-wishers. The media captured a few interviews as the team readied its packs and donned plastic mountaineering boots. An older couple had driven up from Tacoma. Their daughter had just been diagnosed with breast cancer and they wanted to show support. They hiked with us about a hundred yards up the trail. Lou Whittaker and his wife, Ingrid (herself a retired mountain guide), helped with last-minute pack adjustments and saw Peter off on the first leg of what would eventually prove to be his greatest achievement to date.

"What a bonus it was to meet Lou Whittaker," Sue Anne told me. "He watched me struggle to lift my pack up to my knee to get it on my back. 'Don't you want to take some stuff out of that pack?' he asked. He suggested that I at least put my camera inside my pack. I'd rather have given up my water than my camera. My pack rat nature just about got the best of me."

Off Sue Anne went with the trek team, sweat and sunscreen dripping into her eyes. "I couldn't see," she recounts. "Not only that, an hour into the climb, my legs started getting rubbery. I fell behind. I got panicky. 'Holy cow,' I thought, 'I went to all this trouble to get on this team, now what if I don't make it?' I was used to saying in my mind, 'I can do this,' and my body would do it. Maybe I was wrong. Maybe I wasn't cut out for this assignment.

"At one point, on a steep ridge, my heavy pack started throwing me off balance and I suddenly forgot about taking pictures. My total focus was on placing one foot in front of the other and getting across that ridge. Eventually, we all made it across and then plopped down in the snow. No one said a word. No one wanted to admit how sobering that stretch had been. Then I heard someone ask, 'Are we going back the same way?' The guides told us that Aconcagua had many such spans and I had the distinct feeling that they were checking to see if anyone would freak out." No one did. The team was already beginning to show its mettle.

Roberta, however, was still full of doubt. "After the climbing school, which exhausted me, and seeing those ugly slides of Aconcagua, I thought, 'There is no way this is going to hold my attention through the physical strain.' Aconcagua didn't look like a pretty mountain—no forests, no snow, only rock. I was so upset. I didn't want to take myself off the team because all the women were so great. But I thought, 'For the greater goal, I have to take myself off this project. I am the weak link and I'm jeopardizing the trek's success by taking somebody else's place.' I was depressed. I didn't talk to anybody. I simply packed my pack and went to bed. Then I realized, 'If I take myself off the team, I'll have to give back all this great stuff.' I didn't want to do that!

"On the hike to our camp on the Nisqually Glacier, I actually had a good day. There were lots of narrow trails and ridges where you had to pay attention instead of focusing on your pain and suffering. I really liked that focus on the effort. I told myself, 'Okay, I'm still taking myself off the team. This will be my big move—then I'm done.'"

Despite her ups and downs in confidence, Roberta had come a long way from being "the last one chosen for a team" to a full-fledged Expedition Inspiration team member. In June, I had led a climb of 13,053-foot Mount Dana in Yosemite National Park with Roberta, Nancy Johnson, Saskia, Claudia Crosetti, Claudia's father, Vic, and several friends in support. We camped out the night before our climb in Tuolumne Meadows at 9,000 feet, to acclimatize to the higher elevation.

Roberta had been working out for about a month in preparation for Mount Dana. "I had all the wrong gear. I had borrowed a little daypack from a friend, and the only tent I had was huge. Everyone else had these little backpacking tents. The night before we left for Yosemite, I told Saskia, 'I'm not going to date anybody. I'm probably going to be by myself and make my family my focus.'"

Saskia asked, "Why is that?"

"Well, look at me," Roberta said. "I'm thirty-five, I live in the Bay Area—not known as a haven for straight, eligible bachelors—and I've got scars on my chest, my belly, my back. I'm missing a breast. I've had cancer twice and I can't have any children. Who could cope with all that?"

About an hour into the Mount Dana climb, Roberta was hurting. "At the first break, I asked someone how long we had been hiking—an hour! I thought, 'There's no way, *no way,* I can do this.' It was just as in school. I was always the last one coming off the track, panting, my face red and my eyes bulging out, ready to puke any minute. And then I noticed that there were others along without much hiking experience. Francey, one of the more experienced hikers climbing with us, offered to stay back with me. She encouraged me, reminded me to drink water and breathe deeply, to pace myself.

"And then I met Kipp. He was supposed to have been climbing Mount Dana with his girlfriend, but they'd had a fight, so he had come by himself. He started hiking with me and Francey and we started talking. He noticed that I was wearing a Breast Cancer Fund T-shirt, so I told him all about what we were doing and pretty soon we were talking, talking, talking, all the way to the top! When I got to the summit, I wanted to cry, but I didn't want to do that in front of him. Kipp told me later, 'You didn't look like someone who had done this very often.'

"Achieving the summit of Mount Dana was the first time since I had studied dance that I felt physically challenged and successful. That huge mountain gave me such a rush. Kipp showed me how to glissade in the snow on the way down—what a blast! Then I got my boot stuck, wedged between two rocks, and Kipp had to rescue me."

As it turned out, Kipp lived in a neighboring town about a half hour's drive from Roberta. She invited him back to our campsite for dinner that night, where we all toasted each other's success. "At the campfire," says Roberta, "I looked over at Kipp and had the instant premonition that he would be the next man with whom I would be intimate."

At the time of the shakedown climb, Roberta had not yet realized her premonition, but she was working on it. "I hadn't dated in fifteen years. I told Kipp that he could call me once he resolved his situation with his girlfriend. It wasn't until after Rainier that we had our first date."

While the trek team hiked to the Nisqually Glacier, the summit team took a different route, one that led up the Muir Snowfield. Vicki planned to turn back at the rest stop at Pebble Creek, around 7,800 feet. She had invited her friend, Ron Gregg, to climb with us so that she'd have someone to accompany her down the mountain. Ron is the energetic, mountain-climbing founder and president of Outdoor Research, Inc., a company that makes technical gloves, gaiters, hats and a variety of other accessories for mountaineering and other outdoor sports. He had donated expedition gloves and gaiters to the team. At Pebble Creek, Vicki decided to go a little higher.

"I didn't want to turn around," she remembers. "I felt great and wanted to go all the way, but I kept thinking that I needed to save my energy to recover from chemo and train for Aconcagua. I had also told my boss that I'd be back to work the next day."

The other summit team members offered words of encouragement and reassurance to Vicki. She finally decided to turn with Ron at the next rest stop, high on the snowfield at 9,000 feet. She looked exuberant and healthy. This was the first time the team had climbed together and the first time one of us had turned back for any reason. It hurt to bid her good-bye and left many of us wondering who, if anyone, might be the next to turn?

When the trek team reached its campsite on the Nisqually Glacier that afternoon, Sue Anne says she tried to appear as if she were helping out, but, she adds, "I was so tired. I had rarely camped out, and never on snow. When my teammates saw what I had in my pack, they were amazed. I was rightfully labeled a pack rat rather than a backpacker. I wasn't certain what the guides were going to feed us, so I had brought some of my own health foods and extra for anyone else who might want it. I had fresh fruit: two grapefruits, two oranges and three plums. I had granola bars. I even had extra shoes. Nobody else took extra shoes because they knew better. But, later that night, when my tentmates had to go potty, they used my shoes because they were easier to put on than our big mountaineering boots. I also had a clipboard and paper because I thought I'd keep a journal. It seemed I had brought enough for twelve people. One of the guides finally said to me, 'Don't do this anymore. Take care of yourself.' Many cancer patients acknowledge that there is a cancer mentality. We're caretakers, always trying to take care of everybody else, sometimes neglecting ourselves."

In a positive sense, this caretaking tendency was evident among the members of both teams and reinforced the notion of teamwork. The amount of support and nurturing among the survivors was incredible to behold and even spread among the support team members. If one of the climbers needed encouragement, it was readily offered. If a pack got too heavy, another would help carry the load. If somebody needed help setting up a tent or filling water bottles, someone else was there to lend a hand. The guides frequently had to remind the survivors to focus on their own needs first, before helping others.

As soon as the trek team finished setting up its tents, Erika rounded up everyone for a stretching session. As Sue Anne recalls, "The sun had gone behind the ridge by then and I was freezing. Erika got us out there, stretching, moving, getting the blood going. I warmed right up. Being on the glacier on that huge mountain was a wonderful experience. No TV, no radio, great sunsets. It reminded me of Africa in the Peace Corps, where our big entertainment was to run up on top of a nearby rock in the evening and watch the sun go down."

While the women worked out with Erika, Tuck completed a special project. Using his ice ax, he carved a u-shaped table and bench out of the glacial ice, big enough to seat the entire trek team. He covered the bench with foam sleeping pads to keep everyone's bottoms warm, and Roger picked wildflowers and heather on a nearby ridge to decorate the table. There they feasted, talked and laughed until the cold mountain air forced them into their tents for the night.

Before tentmates were chosen, Claudia Crosetti and Nancy Johnson asked the others, "Does anybody snore? If you do, we'd rather not have you in our tent because we're light sleepers." Sue Anne and Devra both claimed not to be snorers and were allowed in the "quiet tent."

Roberta, Nancy Hudson, Kim and Patty clustered together in another tent. Tuck assigned Eleanor and Sara to their own tent. Sara says, "He always treated us special." To Tuck's credit, that comment was made by most of the trek team members. There was no small amount of bonding between Tuck, a nurturing male, and these women. By the time they came off the mountain, they were calling themselves "King Tuck and the Hot Flashers."

At Camp Muir, the summit team had divided into tent teams of Annette and guide Catie; Laura and Saskia; Dr. Bud and Paul; John Cooley, Peter and guide Kurt; Jimmy and Susie; Claudia B-S and me. We ate a hearty one-pot dinner and retired early. Pete planned to sound summit reveille before dawn.

Claudia B-S was also my tentmate on Aconcagua. We bonded immediately upon discovering that we both are "chocoholics." Claudia B-S denied herself the pleasure of chocolate when she wasn't climbing. On the mountain, however, Snickers, Nestle's and Hershey became dietary staples, along with anything else that was put in front of her. "Jim and I mostly eat vegetarian at home," she explained to me, "but on a mountain, you need fuel. Everything tastes good." I would discover later on Aconcagua that Claudia B-S did not suffer the common high-altitude side effect of appetite loss. On the other hand, above 14,000 feet, my craving for chocolate strangely disappeared.

Sometime in the middle of the night, I ventured outside on the snow to answer nature's call and once again marveled at the blanket of stars above. Two months earlier, I had stood atop 19,340-foot Huayna Potosi in Bolivia with Peter and Laura, with the vast crest of the Andes laid out below us, but I had yet to reach the 14,411-foot summit of Mount Rainier. My last two attempts had been thwarted by blizzards on the upper mountain. I knew that if we had good weather and no accidents, I would make it to the summit. I prayed that the weather of the past two days would hold just a day longer. "Please let us reach our goal," I whispered to the mountain gods before climbing back into my warm sleeping bag.

Claudia B-S woke me up in what seemed like seconds later, as she climbed back into the tent.

"Whaaaat?" I groaned.

"Pete got up while I was peeing," she said. "It's time to go." It was three-thirty. We'd have to hustle to get on the trail by five o'clock.

We each gobbled a granola bar, threw down a cup of hot tea and pulled on a warm fleece sweater, outerwear jacket and bib pants over our long underwear. We strapped crampons onto boots, cinched down climbing harnesses, grabbed ice axes and slapped helmets onto heads. After roping together in three different teams, we struck out across the Cowlitz Glacier en route to the summit. We reached our first rest stop at 11,000 feet on the Ingraham Flats, a level slope on the Ingraham Glacier, in time to watch red and yellow fingers of sunlight stretch across the sky and illuminate nearby peaks. The weather was cold but the sky was clear, and we shivered both from the air temperature and in anticipation of the next pitch, which led up the steep nose of a rock- and ice-covered abutment called Disappointment Cleaver. This point had been aptly named by an early climbing party that thought it had reached the summit, to discover, when the clouds cleared, that they had only climbed to 12,500 feet.

Annette was quiet. This was her first foray into the mountains and, although a confident and determined person, she was struggling. "Every time I'd start to feel a little slump," she told me afterward, "I'd think about all the people who were supporting my efforts on this expedition and I'd get a fresh burst of energy. It was an amazing experience." Whenever one of us would ask her, "How're you doing?" she'd nod her head and give us a thumbs-up. She was tough.

The team finally reached the top of the Cleaver, and took another rest break. Saskia had used up most of her energy hauling herself up the route. She was thoroughly dehydrated, badly sunburned from the previous day and exhausted. Peter made the wise decision of asking Kurt Wedburg to guide her back to Camp Muir. We all became very somber, once again feeling distress at watching a team member turn back. Would this happen on Aconcagua? What if no one made it to the summit? Peter quickly encouraged us to focus on eating, drinking and applying sunscreen in preparation for the next stretch.

"Next stop, 13,800 feet," he said. "Once we get going, if anyone has any trouble or feels they can't go on, we won't be able to send another guide back down with you. Instead, we'll put you in a sleeping bag and anchor you to the snow, then pick you up on our way down from the summit."

This is a logical plan on a guided trip, but one that causes nervous gurgling in the pit of the stomach. Nobody wants to be the one who literally gets bagged. Annette later recalled how Peter's statement had motivated her. "I was determined that it would not be me, no way, no how."

~

By the time the summit team reached the top of Disappoint-ment Cleaver, the trek team had awakened to a new revelation: at altitude, certain bodily functions, in particular snoring and flatulence, manifest themselves in ways that might not surface at sea level. That first night, Sue Anne and Devra had revealed themselves to be "marathon snorers," describes Claudia Crosetti. "In the morning, I told Devra, 'Next time somebody asks you if you snore, the answer is a definite, 'Yes, like a buzzsaw!'"

Kim added, "In our tent, we nicknamed Nancy Hudson 'Zip-per' because she sounded like someone opening up a zipper when she snored—*zip, zip, zip*!"

The summit team members already had agreed that Dr. Bud and Paul were appropriate tentmates as both snored "like big dogs," as one woman described them. Another said, "Dr. Bud's lilting refrain was often drowned out by Paul's *basso profundo*."

Of course, everyone suffered flatulence from the combination of extreme exertion and eating rehydrated food, cheese, salami, dried fruit and energy bars. "Now I know why Peter calls his sleeping bag a 'fart sack,'" said another team member. We all learned a first-hand lesson in acceptance. As Lou Whittaker says, "When you spend time in a tent with another person, you have to practice tolerance with all your senses."

That first morning, while the summit team continued its as-cent, the trek team eagerly began its climb from the Nisqually Glacier to Camp Muir, a challenging four-thousand-foot eleva-tion gain. Carrying only a jacket, water, sunscreen, snacks and camera, everyone's pack was lighter than on the previous day—except Erika's. She was carrying a big surprise for the summit team.

Roberta thought of turning around several times. "Jen and Erika stayed back with me," she recalls. "They kept talking to me, encouraging me. The only way I could keep going was to think in terms of rhythm and music. I'd do a sort of swing with my poles and arms, focusing on the movement."

Without the excess weight she had been carrying in her pack, Sue Anne enjoyed an easier hike to Camp Muir. "For me, reaching 10,000 feet was a big triumph," she says. "I finally got into rest-stepping and pressure breathing, oxygenating myself. I finally *got* it and it felt wonderful!"

For Roberta, the last few hundred feet up the snowfield to Camp Muir was the hardest. "I thought 'This is never going to end. I'm going to die on this bloody mountain!' But, I finally made it. I was so exhausted and exasperated, I sat there and said to myself, 'Big deal.' Then I looked up and saw the other mountains out there, the immense vista, and I started bawling. Patty and Kim came over to me and we all stood there, hugging each other and crying with joy. It was such a relief. It was at that moment that I told myself, 'You have to do this.' All my life, I have told myself that I cannot do things and watched my life pass me by. I could not let myself do that again. I thought, 'If I do nothing else in my life, I have to do this.' Then I started shaking, got a blistering headache and went sheet-white. Devra was the first to notice and hustled me into the hut. Sue Anne came in and started rubbing my hands, my arms, trying to get some circulation going, applying acupressure.

"I had never really sweated from extreme exertion before. I guess I became dehydrated on the hike to Muir. I drank more water and began to feel better. Devra told the guides that I wasn't feeling well, so Jen and Erika came to see me. Erika said, 'You used up all your reserves. Drink more water. You'll be all right.' Later, after we got down off the mountain, Erika said, 'Your body had no business being up there. You hiked up there on your mind alone. Your body was shutting down; you had nothing left.' I had never pushed myself like that before. I was proud of myself."

The rest of the trek team made it to Camp Muir in good form. Sara says she felt more mentally scared than anything. "Learning the ice ax arrest the first day scared me witless. But, you know, that's okay. I learned it. You do it. I think the most frightened I've ever been in this context was the first time I had to cross a suspension bridge in Nepal four years before on a trip with Fritz. That really terrified me. The bridge is merely hanging above the river, you know. I didn't think I'd be able to do it, but I had to. It's hard focusing your mind like that the first time. And, the older you get, the more fearful you become. Thirteen suspension bridges later, I was doing fine. Rainier was the same way. You can make yourself scared. You have to overcome the fear."

The summit team reached its last rest stop at 13,800 feet while the trek team was still hiking toward Camp Muir. Peter kept the breaks short, ten to fifteen minutes at most, so that we wouldn't cool down entirely and lose body heat. Even with a clear, sunny sky, the temperature was about twenty degrees with a brisk breeze that made the air feel colder. Claudia B-S was wearing her ever present grin. If she felt pain, she ignored it. Laura looked calm and confident, having summited Rainier several times in previous years. Annette looked cold, but she was grinning, too. I suddenly realized that we were *all* grinning. The summit of Mount Rainier, only forty-five minutes away, was surely ours this day.

As we rounded the summit ridge, the wind picked up, but we leaned into it and plunged ahead, step by step, breath by breath. For me, the anticipation of setting foot on the summit of Rainier after four thwarted attempts was nearly overwhelming. I had to suppress tears so that I could continue to pressure breathe. I could only imagine how Annette, a complete novice, felt. Later, she told me, "Cold, I felt cold. I began to appreciate the experience once we started back down and I began to warm up. Then I realized, I really *like* mountain climbing!"

One by one, we gained the summit. We hugged, whooped, hollered and thanked God that no one had to be bagged. The wind had whipped up on top, but the view was magnificently clear. We could see boats on Puget Sound, and all surrounding and distant peaks, including Mount Baker, Mount Adams, Mount Saint Helens and, to the south in Oregon, Mount Hood. Catie, John, Susie and Paul huddled with Annette while Peter, Laura, Claudia B-S, Dr. Bud, Jimmy and I hiked across the snow-filled, three-mile-square crater to the summit register. There we watched as Laura recorded the momentous occasion. Expedition Inspiration had achieved the first leg of its goal.

I wrote a thank you in the register to Lou and Peter for introducing me to mountain climbing, and I added special notes to my mother and to my partner, Francey. After so many attempts, I wanted to make sure I did it right, in case my journeys never led here again.

A little past noon, as the trek team reached Camp Muir, the summit team was well into its descent. When we emerged atop the last ridge before the descent to Camp Muir, we paused to look for signs of our teammates. Suddenly, we heard a cry echo across the glacier: "Ya-a-a-a-y!" The trek team! They had climbed up onto nearby Muir Peak with the intent of spotting us. We quickly sent back a cheer: "Ya-a-a-a-y!" Cheers and tears and energy filled the expanse between us and propelled us the last mile into camp. There our teammates surrounded us with hugs, laughter and excited chatter. Then Erika presented her surprise: a giant, juicy watermelon, which disappeared in a matter of minutes.

After spending another beautifully clear night on the mountain, both teams descended and reunited at the Paradise Inn to celebrate. Laura and Pete declared the shakedown a success and proudly pronounced us "a team." On the mountain, we had formed a bond that would now carry us through to Aconcagua. Laura was one step closer to realizing her dream, which now had become our dream, too.

At that point, Roberta tearfully confessed her original intent to quit the team. "But I can't, I won't," she added, fighting back sobs. "This was my summit. If I do nothing else, this will always be my summit."

Claudia B-S announced, "This was my first cancer-free moment since I was diagnosed. From here, I want to move away from the disease, toward wellness."

We roared our approval. We toasted each other. We thanked Laura and Peter for their dedication and perseverance. We thanked the guides for their patience, help and advice. We thanked the Lord, we thanked Buddha, we thanked every deity that might be watching over our little corner of the world. In only six months, we'd be heading to another corner of the world to climb Aconcagua. God willing, we'd all stay healthy and strong until then.

The next morning, the team awoke at the Nisqually Lodge to gray skies and dark clouds converging on Mount Rainier. The mountain was showing off again.

Part Two

The Inward Journey

"You do your best, and then you let go ...let go of knowing the outcome beforehand." —Annette Porter

Discovery

AFTER THE SHAKEDOWN CLIMB, the team returned home infused with a greater sense of unity and purpose, and a commitment to training that intensified during the five months leading up to the expedition. Individual training routines varied but generally included climbing hills, stairs or bleachers while wearing a thirty- to forty-pound backpack to strengthen legs, plus running, fitness walking or bicycling to build cardiovascular strength and endurance. Many of the women added a weight workout at a gym for overall conditioning and to build additional muscle.

Several of the team members conditioned by climbing. Late in the summer, Vicki, Claudia B-S, Sue Anne and Roberta climbed 12,264-foot Matterhorn Peak in the Sierra Nevadas. In the fall, Annette climbed two volcanic peaks in Mexico: 17,887-foot Popocatepetl and 18,701-foot Orizaba. Laura had already climbed them that spring. Eleanor and Sara met in Aspen, Colorado, to climb in the Rockies and work out with a personal trainer. Kipp assigned himself as Roberta's personal trainer, and accompanied her on outings nearly every weekend.

Each team member understood that strength and endurance would be key factors to success—as would a healthy dose of what Peter called "PMA," for Positive Mental Attitude. All the breast cancer survivors were well acquainted with the power of PMA. In many instances, PMA was all that had gotten them through their diagnoses and courses of treatment.

After the shakedown climb, media exposure increased. In hometown newspapers, the national press and on TV, each survivor's story was told and retold. As the tale of each woman's journey through breast cancer unfolded, a strong message was sent out to the American public: be vigilant in your health care; get second opinions; take charge of your life.

Laura Evans had always "taken charge." At age forty, when she was diagnosed, she was accustomed to success, to getting what she wanted, no matter how much effort it took. Sexy, active, creative, infused with a wild and crazy spirit that propelled her fast-paced lifestyle, she charged exuberantly through each day. Breast cancer was the only roadblock that had ever stopped her. And then, it only stopped her momentarily before she took charge again, but at a different pace.

"I made a lot of changes," she told me. "I learned that change is the only absolute and it's the hardest thing to do. But an illness like cancer forces you to change. You tend to temper your expectations—of yourself and others. From the moment of your diagnosis and then on, you start learning to focus on the moment."

The actualization of living in the moment is not something that comes over breast cancer patients—or any cancer patient—

at a set time during the course of the disease. There is no standard formula for dealing with breast cancer. Not all tumors are pea-sized lumps. Not all mammograms are one hundred percent reliable. Each person's experience differs, depending on the type of breast cancer, its stage of development, the doctor's philosophy regarding surgery and treatment, the person's age and situation (Do you have insurance? Do you have someone to help care for you?). A look at each team member's experience with breast cancer reveals a significant dichotomy between general information from the medical community and what happens in real life.

When Kim O'Meara Anderson's three-month-old son, Evan, began rejecting her left breast, Kim's OB/GYN doctor first believed that she might have a clogged milk duct.

"I really owe my diagnosis to Evan," says Kim. "If he hadn't had difficulty nursing, I wouldn't have had the suspicion. During pregnancy, your breasts change so much. Mine were like two footballs, so engorged that it was impossible to really detect anything abnormal. And breast cancer is not something you think about during pregnancy."

Kim adds, "I knew that milk ducts were vertical, like a section of an orange. Instead of being a vertical section, this mass was stretching horizontally across my breast and under my arm. I became really alarmed. Evan's pediatrician finally made the connection that it might be something other than a clogged duct."

Kim stubbornly refused to stop nursing. She wanted to keep their routine as normal as possible for Evan. "I could have a sonogram or ultrasound but not a mammogram because it would contaminate the breast milk," she says. "Finally, in March, they got a needle biopsy. Up until then, the doctors had been having trouble getting anything out of the mass.

"They stuck the needle in and as this dark gray stuff filled the syringe, I'll never forget the look on the doctor's face. I knew, deep down then and there, that it was probably cancer.

"A couple of weeks later, on April 1, I got the pathology report. My general practitioner called and I remember thinking, 'This is just a bad April Fool's Day joke. I'll go to bed tonight and wake up tomorrow and everything will be fine, *la-de-dah-de-dah*.' But it wasn't. The doctor gave me a scary prognosis. They were shocked by the size of the cancer and how quickly it had grown. That's why they classified it Stage 2. I ran the gamut of emotions, from being in denial to thinking the worst. I realized I might not see Evan reach his first birthday."

Ashley Sumner-Cox had recently reached her eighteenth birthday when she first visited her doctor to talk about a breast reduction. She could hardly say "the 'B' word," she says, "especially with my dad sitting there. The doctor asked me, 'What can we do for you?' I was disappearing in my chair. Now I'll shout '*Breast!*' at the top of my lungs. I don't care anymore. Now I'm desensitized. But back then it was very embarrassing, very difficult.

"The doctor examined me and agreed that my breasts were definitely too big for my frame. He said he'd reduce them to a size that would work for me. I thought that was really cool. I did it over Christmas break when no one at school would know. But, of course, they knew. A lot of people just thought I'd lost a lot of weight over the break—which I did, surgically. My mom made the mistake of telling one of my teachers and word got around. That was embarrassing, too."

The doctor called Ashley in early, supposedly to remove her stitches. "The doctor took out all my stitches and it hurt like hell and I wanted to pass out because I couldn't stand the pain," says Ashley. "Ever since then, I've hated pain. Before then, I could take it. I was tough.

"Afterwards, he sat us down and explained what they had found. He told us that he'd sent my breast tissue all over the country to different specialists. He couldn't believe that he had found cancer in an eighteen-year-old. It didn't make sense. But every specimen came back, 'Yes, in fact, this is cancer.' And he said this is reportable because I'm so young. I wish I could get my story published in every medical journal there is because I'd like people to know that, yeah, there is the possibility. You're never too young.

"The cancer was intraductal carcinoma *in situ*, which means, technically, you could call it precancerous. I could have carried it into my thirties or it could have started to metastasize and killed me in a year.

"So we heard this. And my mom began to cry. I was trying not to cry because I was worried about Mom. This big old blow, you know, 'Your daughter has cancer.' And I was saying, 'Well, oka-a-a-a-y.' I had tears in my eyes. I didn't want to cry in front of my mom. I wanted to be tough. So I drove home from the doctor's office because my mom was really upset.

"All I remember the doctor saying was, 'A mastectomy is the best way to go with this. We can do it in the summertime.' It was January and I said, 'No, I want it done now.' Actually, I think the first thing I said was, 'You mean I'm going to have to have more stitches?' I tried to keep a little humor going but it was really, really hard."

$\sim$

It wasn't as hard for sixty-year-old Sara Hildebrand. In August 1993, she had read an article in the *New York Times* about breast cancer. She had been surprised that the paper would show a photo of a mastectomy. She discussed the article with her husband, Fritz, a pulmonologist at the La Salle Clinic, near their home in Neenah, Wisconsin.

Sara recalls: "I said to Fritz, 'Okay, we're down to it. It says the risk is one out of nine. What happens to me if I get it? Where would you like to see me go and who would do the surgery?' He had it all figured out by the time I finished asking my questions. He said I would go to the same hospital his patients go to. He gave me the name of the physician he would recommend, someone we'd known for thirty years."

The next morning, Sara was scheduled to have her routine annual physical exam and mammogram. Three days later, she was called back for re-examination by a surgeon. "I had never felt anything during self-examination," Sara says. "But my gynecologist said that the radiologist had seen a shadow that was not there twelve months beforehand. The surgeon didn't feel anything, but suggested that we do a stereotactic biopsy. He said, 'I'm sure it will be negative, Sara, so don't worry about it.' Of course, it was cancer. So then I had all my blood work done and made an appointment for a mastectomy. Got the wheels rolling according to the plan Fritz had laid out for me a couple of weeks before."

Unlike Sara, Eleanor Davis knew that there definitely was a lump in her breast, but it had come and gone with her menstrual period for about a year. "I told my gynecologist about it, but because it would go away after each period, she told me not to worry. Then, one day in April 1979, I was playing tennis and my bra felt really uncomfortable because of the lump. This time, I went to a surgeon for an aspiration biopsy. He also told me, 'Don't worry. You're too young to have breast cancer. I'm sure it will be nothing.' I was forty. A week later, my doctor called to tell me that I had a malignant tumor—tubular carcinoma—in my breast. My husband wasn't home at the time. I walked around the house like a zombie, trying to finish everything up for the day, having nowhere to go with the news."

As soon as her husband, Hal, came home, they scheduled an appointment with a surgeon. "Right off, I told him, 'I want reconstruction,'" says Eleanor. "He said, 'Oh, nobody does that.' Well, that turned me off. I decided to go to another doctor."

Dr. Francis E. Rosato, Chief of Surgery at Thomas Jefferson University Hospital in Philadelphia, finally laid out a plan for Eleanor: a mastectomy, a year of chemotherapy and then reconstruction. Chemotherapy was prescribed because seven lymph nodes were involved.

Eleanor's first instinct was to protect her family. "I didn't want my husband and children to worry about me," she says. "I had a good friend who had died of lung cancer the year before. The children had seen her go through the whole decline and demise and I know they were worried about me with cancer. So my persona through this whole thing was 'I'm okay, I'm strong and I'm going to get through this. I'm not going to have any problems and I don't need any help or support'—which now I realize is crazy. But when you're faced with your own mortality and you have small children, everything else falls by the wayside. You really want to see them grow up. And you want to be the one to raise them."

Patty Duke says she had no worries at all when she went in for her annual physical in October 1992. "When the nurse examined my breasts and asked me, 'Have you ever felt this lump before?' I said, 'Wha-a-a-a-t? Huh? Where?' I didn't feel a pea-sized lump like they use in demonstrations. Instead, I felt a ridge in the upper right side of my right breast and another ridge toward my armpit. I thought, 'How in the world did I miss this?'

"When the nurse ran out to get the doctor, the disbelief and shock began. Dr. Dudley felt the mass and said, 'Well, you're usually lumpy. Let's order another mammogram.' I'd had a mammogram two years before. So, they scheduled me for another one, twenty days from then. They were the longest twenty days of my life. I waited, and waited, and felt the lump. It began to talk to me: 'Hello, I'm here and I'm not going away.' And it began to hurt."

That evening after the mammogram, Dr. Dudley called Patty to tell her that something had shown up on both breasts. "My heart sank," she says. "The next day, they tried to do a needle biopsy but couldn't get anything, so they scheduled me for a bilateral biopsy. The day after that, my husband, Peter, left on a business trip and I received another call from Dr. Dudley that evening. 'Well, kid,' he began, and I knew then. A doctor doesn't call up in the evening and say, 'Well, kid,' unless he has bad news. I had cancer in one breast; the other breast was okay. Shock, disbelief, anger. He said, 'It's tubular cancer, very rare, but it doesn't spread.'

"Dr. Dudley made an appointment for me with an oncologist in Denver. She was of no help at all. She visited with me a few minutes, kept looking at my chart to remind herself who I was and why I was there. Then she told me that I had two choices, a lumpectomy or a mastectomy. I thought, 'Tell me something I don't know.' I needed better help than this. At the time, mastectomies weren't done in Steamboat Springs, which meant I'd have to go to Denver, three hours from home. I might as well have been in New York.

"My mom, who lives in Buffalo, New York, where I grew up, suggested that I come home and see Dr. Cooper, a family friend who also happens to be an oncologist. Peter made plans to fly home early from his business trip to stay with the kids, but I had to leave for Buffalo right away to meet the doctor. It was very difficult leaving Ben and Ryan. It was Ryan's tenth birthday. When I told him about my cancer, he said, 'Tubular cancer? Does that mean it's cool?'—*tubular* being the slang word for *cool* at the time. I said, 'I suppose it is the coolest since I can have it taken out and then it will be all gone.' My older son, Ben, wanted to know if I'd lose my hair. That was *not* cool for a mom. He also asked if I would die. These are all sobering thoughts as you face your children and wonder for how long you really are packing your bags."

Patty left the boys with friends for the night. Peter would be home the following day. "When I dropped off Ryan, I asked my friend Linda, 'Could you please make him a birthday cake?' and then I started to cry again. I felt terrible as a mom, but I think the kids looked at this as an adventure, spending the night with friends on a school night."

For Patty, going home to Buffalo was both frightening and comforting. "My mother was seventy-nine and is the most wonderful person on earth. She is always doing for others, never has an unkind word for anyone, always supportive. To return home and sleep in my old bedroom gave me a sense of security and warmth. I could concentrate on me and what I had to do to get well, to live, and then later I could get back to my boys—Peter, Ben and Ryan—and our dog, Ewik, and take care of them."

In Buffalo, Patty saw Dr. Cooper—or 'Coop,' as the family called him—right away. "He explained all the surgical procedures, how they remove either part or all of the breast," says Patty, "what chemotherapy and radiation are all about. He cleared up many questions, but still left the main one up to me: lumpectomy or mastectomy? I think I had read Dr. Susan Love's *Breast Book* twenty times, but I couldn't make the decision. I met with Dr. Milch, who was to be my surgeon. He had operated on my dad a few years back. I spoke to him of my dilemma and asked him what he would do if he were in my position. He said, 'If you were my wife, I'd ask you to remove the whole breast.' He explained should cancer return to the same breast, it is very difficult to deal with and more difficult to get rid of the second time. That cinched it. A mastectomy it would be. He scheduled the surgery for November 24."

Vicki Boriack's boyfriend discovered the lump in her breast one evening in August 1993. "He guided my hand to the spot and I felt something like a little pea, really deep in my breast," says Vicki. "Of course, I went for a mammogram as soon as possible. Nothing showed up. The radiologist did an ultrasound and said it was just a fibroid and to come back in six months.

"I didn't like living with the lump, so I called my gynecologist, who's a friend, and asked her to look at the report. About three weeks later, she called and said that she wanted me to see a breast surgeon. Because the mammogram also had shown microcalcifications, which can be precancerous, and because the report was 'on the fence,' she felt that further investigation was necessary.

"About a month later, in September, I went to a surgeon, who said, 'Well, it really looks benign, but you have these microcalcifications that I think we need to keep an eye on.' The mammogram I'd had a year and a half before also showed the microcalcifications and they hadn't changed. The surgeon said that if they didn't change in the next six months, he'd do a biopsy. I asked, 'What are the chances of the microcalcifications going away in six months if they've been there for a year-and-a-half?' 'Pretty slim,' he answered. I urged him to do the biopsy right away. I believed it was benign; I had no reason to be afraid. I scheduled the biopsy for the end of October, when my work schedule would slow a bit."

Larry had been Vicki's best friend and lover for several years, although they did not live together. He saw her through her cancer journey. "When I had the biopsy, Larry went with me," says Vicki. "It was a Friday. On Monday, I was pulled out of a meeting at work to take a call from my doctor. He told me I had two kinds of cancer in my breast. The malignant lump, which they removed, was infiltrating ductile cancer and the microcalcifications were *in situ* cancer, confined to the milk ducts. The doctor asked me, 'Do you want me to tell you more or do you want to come in?' I said, 'I think I should come in.' I hung up, sat there for a second and started to hyperventilate. Then I walked to my boss Ken's office and just looked at him. He asked, 'What's wrong?' I said, 'I have cancer.' And I started to cry. Ken put his arms around me and I sobbed. He drove me to the doctor and I called Larry and he met me there.

"Larry and I sat in the doctor's office, holding hands and asking questions. Larry looked devastated. The doctor basically told me that I had two options, a lumpectomy or a mastectomy. He gave me a newsprint pamphlet. I asked to see a picture of a mastectomy, but he didn't have one. I asked if he could give me a list of books to read, but he didn't have that, either. I asked for names of people to talk to and he didn't have any. He rattled off a ton of statistics, but until more tests were complete we wouldn't know where I fit in the numbers.

"He sent me to talk to a medical oncologist and a radiation

oncologist. The radiation oncologist explained what the procedure would be if I had a lumpectomy. The medical oncologist gave me his opinion on whether I should have a lumpectomy or mastectomy based on the type of cancer I had.

"I also attended a Comprehensive Breast Clinic at Stanford. Twelve different oncologists examined me, looked at my test and biopsy results and then argued my case for about an hour and a half. A woman doctor who was one of the head breast surgeons at Stanford insisted that I have a mastectomy. Her opinion won out because of the microcalcifications called DCIS—ductal carcinoma *in situ*—and the fact that they didn't know how extensive they were. If I had a lumpectomy, the cancer could come back."

Vicki's biggest worry was how to tell her kids, Katy and Jonathan. A friend told her, "Just be honest with them. Kids know when you're covering up." On the day she received her biopsy results, she waited until they got home from school. Then she sat down on the floor with them, held hands, and said, "I got my biopsy results back and I have cancer."

They started crying, and Jonathan asked, "Are you going to die?"

Vicki said, "Not if I can help it. I'm going to fight this all the way but it's not going to be easy. I'm going to need a lot of help from you guys to get through this."

According to Vicki, at first the kids didn't ask questions. "Then they started to want to know more. We called their dad and he said the most inappropriate thing: 'If anything happens to your mom, you can come live with me.' He didn't want them to be afraid that they were alone. But it was the absolute wrong thing to say at that time. I thought, we're talking survival here, not death.

"I called my parents to tell them and it was so hard, because the day I learned I had cancer I realized that there was only one thing worse and that would be to hear that one of my children had cancer. My cousin's little boy had been recently diagnosed with cancer. I thought, 'I'll take this any day, if it keeps either of my children from having cancer.'"

A friend steered Vicki to the American Cancer Society and to a local organization called WomenCARE. From both, Vicki collected a pile of reading material. "I couldn't sleep, so I figured I might as well read. Knowledge became a way of fighting back. I read everything I could find printed on breast cancer. I called the oncologist and told him, 'I need more stuff; I don't care if it's over my head.' He loaned me medical books and I bought a medical dictionary. I learned a lot. The more I learned, the more clinical I became, which helped distance me from the fear."

Ultimately, Vicki chose a mastectomy. The choice of lumpectomy involved radiation and Vicki didn't like the potential of the cancer returning in fifteen to twenty years as the result of radiation treatment. "When I called my doctor and told him of my decision, he became real quiet. I asked, 'What's wrong?' He said, 'It's just that I hate doing mastectomies on young women.' I was thirty-nine. I wanted to grow old, get wrinkles and see my grandchildren. I felt that a mastectomy would give me that opportunity."

Nancy Hudson, also a young single mother, lives in Marin County, California, an area that has one of the highest incidences of breast cancer in the nation, and, consequently, some of the best treatment facilities. Unfortunately, Nancy did not happen to visit one of them initially.

Nancy had helped care for a close friend who had recently had a mastectomy and who urged Nancy to get a mammogram.

"I finally agreed and went to an imaging center in a shopping mall," says Nancy. "They told me I had microcalcifications and to come back the next day for another mammogram. I did. And they said, 'Oh, don't worry. It's the same thing we saw yesterday. Forget about it.'

"I had an intuition that something was not right in my body. So I called my stepfather, a thoracic surgeon in Columbus, Ohio. I flew to Columbus on a Tuesday and he scheduled me with one of his colleagues for a regular biopsy that Thursday. After the biopsy, I was shopping with my mother at my grandfather's store and they called us there to tell me that the biopsy had revealed interductal carcinoma. My mother started crying and said, 'Why couldn't it have been me?'"

Nancy had little time for the news to settle in, or to explore options. "On the following Tuesday, I went in for surgery," she says. "I signed a paper that read that if they found another primary site, I'd agree to a mastectomy rather than a lumpectomy. I woke up without a breast.

"It was over like that. My stepfather had insisted that I get the surgery done that week. In his mind, the minute you get cancer, you cut it out and it's a done deal. After the surgery, I was recuperating at their house and he caught me crying. He said, 'Quit crying. You could be dead.' I was overwhelmed at what had happened and how quickly it had all happened. I was upset about my marriage and I missed my boys. But my stepfather shows very little consideration for the emotional aspects of life. I was glad when I was able to leave and get home to my children."

Sue Anne also had a premonition that she might have cancer. She was in the kitchen one morning when it happened. "I remember a funny feeling had come over me and at the same time a thought had come to me: 'I wonder if I have cancer?' It was as though someone had tapped me on the shoulder. I knew my breasts were lumpy, but I didn't know what they should feel like.

"Both my husband and I had been dealing with depression for a couple of years. The depression had separated us within our own house. On the surface, I carried on, but I could feel myself disintegrating. I had told Gary that if we didn't do something about our situation, I was afraid it would manifest itself physically.

"It took nearly four months to get an appointment for a mammogram, late that summer. Afterward, the doctor referred me to a surgeon. I thought, 'Good grief—a surgeon, me?' I had never had surgery, rarely had I been sick. The surgeon looked at the mammogram and examined me and said, 'There appear to be some calcifications. Watch your breasts. If anything changes, let me know.' Gary had had a bout with melanoma right after we married. A mole had turned black. They cut it out, monitored the site every three months for several years, then every six months. The doctors were very vigilant with him. So when my doctor said, 'Watch it and let me know if there are changes,' I didn't think anything of it.

"That was in September 1989. Three years later, in December I went in for a follow-up. My nipple was oozing. There was redness as well as pus and that alarmed me. A hard, little, BB-sized lump also had shown up. I knew that wasn't right and I started reading everything I could find. I went to a couple of doctors before one finally said, 'We'd better biopsy that.'

"When I finally went in for a biopsy on February 9, 1993, the doctor looked at my records and said, 'I see here in 1989 you were seen by a surgeon and you were supposed to go back in three months.' 'What?' I exclaimed. I knew I would not have forgotten. I couldn't believe it. Nobody had monitored me as they had my husband. Somehow I had slipped through the cracks of my HMO.

"During my pre-op visit with the surgeon, I had to remind him that I was the one with the oozing nipple, BB-sized lump and calcifications. He seemed distant and distracted. I assumed that he was overworked or burned out.

"After the biopsy, I realized that I had to start taking charge of my illness. I decided to have a local anesthetic for the biopsy. The doctors told me that usually wasn't done, but I persisted and they eventually agreed. I had given birth to both my daughters at home with no medication. The anesthesiologist and pre-op team thought that was unusual. That's when I realized that their frame of reference was different from mine. I was more into a holistic lifestyle, natural medicine and vegetarianism. But I had never been faced with a life-threatening illness.

"The anesthesiologist told me to let him know if I needed more anesthesia. They numbed my breast. I had arranged to have some tapes playing and I practiced deep breathing. I did not feel full of fear. I could smell the cauterization and hear the cutting. I breathed deeply and tried to stay centered.

"As the assistant surgeon was sewing me up, I asked the anesthesiologist, 'Did he get three samples?' The anesthesiologist responded, 'Well, it looks like one.' I said, 'Tell him he was supposed to take three.' Then the thought came over me, 'Maybe it's like you sometimes hear, when they open you up the cancer is so vast that they close you up again, a hopeless case.' For the first time, the seriousness of this chapter of my life began to creep in.

"I was in the recovery room, the only one wide awake. Everyone else was still doped up. Eventually, the surgeon came in.

'You had a question about your surgery?' I asked him if he had taken three samples. He hesitated. 'Well.' I said, 'You told me you were going to sample the oozing cyst, the calcifications and the lump.' He finally admitted, 'I forgot.'

"I was furious. 'You forgot? I can't believe you *forgot*.' I had this overwhelming feeling of 'Why me?' He started to say, 'We can reschedule—' and I said, 'What, and go through all this again?' I could feel the nervous presence of the nurses and anesthesiologist in the room. They knew this was a boner. The whole room could hear the discussion. My nurse and anesthesiologist were being very nice. The surgeon finally said, 'We can wheel you back in and open you up again.' And they did."

This time, Sue Anne didn't listen to her tapes. She talked to the surgeon. "I know they can tell right away even though they make you wait a week or two for results, so I asked him, 'What do you think?' He wouldn't commit. I looked up into the mirror above me and was surprised to see that it was dirty and full of smudges. I said, 'I can see why you put people under, so they don't ask too many questions.' When he was finished, I asked him, 'Do you know what my name is?' He had to look at my chart.

"Confidence in my care was waning and I needed all my energy to cope with my emotions. I began to realize that I'd have to muster some assertiveness to get better care. The doctor's nonchalant attitude was not comforting, and was a real shock—I mean, it was *my body* he was being nonchalant about.

"I decided to document the whole episode and file a complaint. I took the complaint to Patient Assistance and asked for a new doctor. I got jostled around there, too. I wanted a referral to the nearby university medical center, but they told me they couldn't do that.

"Then I remembered that a friend's husband was a doctor at

an associated facility. I discovered he was the chief surgeon, so I made an appointment with him. At last, I felt I had a human being I could relate to—a friend, even.

"As it turned out, the first sample, the cyst, was precancerous. It was the second sample, the BB-sized lump, that was the culprit. If I had not been awake and alert to the situation, they would have missed it.

"The new surgeon recommended a mastectomy. Although the lump wasn't that big, they had classified it as Stage 2 infiltrating ductile carcinoma. I struggled with the emotional disbelief that this was happening to me. I read everything about lumpectomies and mastectomies. Losing the breast wasn't as big a trauma for me as dealing with my level of medical care.

"I had a mastectomy in February, a couple of weeks after the biopsy. Then I was sent to an oncologist. Because seven of twelve lymph nodes were involved, four weeks after surgery I was scheduled to begin chemotherapy, followed by radiation.

"I felt like a little kid in the oncologist's office. The chair was very low and his desk very high. The doctor sat in a high-backed, thronelike chair. On his desk were two eight-by-ten picture frames blocking my view of him. The psychological situation was not optimum. He asked if I had any questions. I asked, 'Could we move these?' as I scooted one of the photos over a couple of inches. He left the photo in its new spot, but he was definitely affronted. He started telling me about different trials, protocols, and which chemotherapy did I want? I hated the idea of chemo, so I asked, 'Do you have any experimental alternative treatments?' I've always trusted my intuitions, but I was feeling overwhelmed by the wrath of fear in everyone else surrounding me. I didn't have the support, energy or funding to make Deepak Chopra my physician, so I tried to figure out how to make the best of this situation. I listened to Chopra's tapes. If he had said, 'Do chemo,'

I'd have done it without hesitation. I really struggled. I carried a card with me that read, 'Grow where you're planted.' I decided to take the chemo and do my best to grow with the situation."

Annette Porter also feared chemotherapy. "That was the big horror of all the treatments," she says. "I had randomly qualified for a protocol that called for the highest dosage of Adriamycin that I could tolerate. I also had done my own research and it looked like the right way to go. Adriamycin was deemed to be one of the most effective breast cancer drugs, although it could have dangerous side effects. It was really a leap of faith."

Annette was thirty-two when she discovered a lump in her right breast during a self-examination in February 1991. She had a mammogram followed by a biopsy. "I was at work and I received a voice mail message from my gynecologist asking me to call her and have her interrupted. When I called she was delivering a baby so I didn't have her interrupted, but I was thinking, 'This is bad news because I am supposed to interrupt her. I should've gotten a post card in the mail, not a phone call.'

"I asked a friend of mine at work to sit in my office with me while I called the doctor again. My friend knew I'd had the biopsy. This time, I had the doctor interrupted. She said, 'I don't know how to tell you this.' I responded, 'You have to tell me. Just tell me.' She said, 'Well, we think it's cancer. There are suspicious cells in there.' I asked, 'Well, do you *think* it's cancer or do you know for sure?' She finally said, 'There *are* cancerous cells. They are not suspicious cells.'

"My initial reaction was to go numb, then flood with emotion and cry. I was glad my friend was there.

"When I finally turned my attention back to the doctor, I asked her for some names of doctors to see. She said, 'I really think you are going to want someone as blunt as you are, so here's so-and-so.' She gave me several names. One of the doctors could squeeze me in that day, so I went.

"This visit was to be a consultation, of course, but I said to him, 'Take it out. I don't want to wait two weeks. You can't ask me to walk around with this in my body. Get it *out*.' The doctor said, 'No, it's important that you make the right decision for yourself.' I said, 'Great. Take it out.' He was patient and got me started in the right direction."

In interviewing different doctors, Annette recalls that it became her "little test" to be able to be on a first-name basis with them. "One doctor was real bothered by this," she remembers. "Finally, I told him this wasn't going to work. I said, 'I can call you Dr. Blah, but then you would need to address me as Miss Porter, and since we're talking about injecting lethal poisons into my body, I'd like to be on a more intimate basis with my doctor.' I ended up with Peter, my oncologist, and Rick, my surgeon, but not before I had traveled to six different doctors. I was looking for the 'right' diagnosis," says Annette, "and for a smart doctor who would tell me that the others were dumb. I didn't want to believe that I had cancer. I even flew my own slides and test results down to Houston, Texas, to the M.D. Anderson Cancer Center. I figured no one would get the results mixed up if I took them myself. I kept thinking, 'Boy, somebody's made a *big* mistake here.' The doctor at M.D. Anderson not only confirmed it was cancer, but also informed me that it was one of the worst kinds: invasive ductal cancer. While the lump was small, it was very aggressive and had already spread to my lymph nodes.

"Initially, I thought that this meant imminent death. My uncle had died the year before of lung cancer. I had watched him go through the transformation from healthy to sick to dead, all in a matter of months. I kept telling myself, 'But, I don't *look* sick like Uncle Jack.' Sitting in the lobby at M.D. Anderson, I saw all sorts of cancer patients, some pushing their IVs along, one with a mechanical voice box. 'I am not one of these people,' I repeated to myself. 'I do not want to join this club.' Of course, once I decided to be part of it, I realized it's really a wonderful club. But I certainly entered kicking and screaming."

Mary Yeo had found a lump in her left breast in March 1988. "The doctor who read my mammogram said that it didn't show anything significant, and recommended another one in six months. So in September, I had another mammogram and this time a mass appeared in my right breast. The doctor decided to do a needle biopsy. The surgeon put three wires into my breast, all pointing toward the lump, and then withdrew a sample from the lump. It was really painful and felt as though he were pulling the whole inside of my breast to the outside.

"My doctor is a straightforward, no-bones-about-it type of guy. I walked into his office a couple of days later and he said, 'Mary, I have bad news for you. You have breast cancer.' Boom! My jaw dropped down and my eyes popped open. The cancer was in my right breast. I had never felt anything there. The lump in the left breast turned out to be a calcification.

"My oldest daughters, Kathy and Mary, were with me," says Mary. "They were with me all the time, for every doctor visit, for surgery. I'm sure they started thinking about it themselves. Every so often I'd break down and start crying and one or more of my sons or daughters would be there, hugging me, reassuring me that everything was okay. My daughter Mary is a nurse, and she brought me all sorts of reading material so that I could learn what my chances and options were and where I stood.

"I was lucky to catch the cancer early. It was intraductal and pre-Stage One. I could have had a lumpectomy, but I chose a mastectomy and never considered reconstruction. I guess at fifty-three I was past the age of vanity. Luckily, no lymph nodes were involved, so I didn't have to undergo chemo or radiation. The other positive thing that happened at that time was the birth of my grandson Daniel, two days before my surgery."

The night before Mary was to go to the hospital, her daughter Carol stayed with her. While dressing for bed, Mary had "a great idea," she recollects. "I called Carol into my room and asked her to draw a smiley face on my breast. She drew some nice eyes and the smile and then I told her, 'You don't need to add the nose—it's already there!' We got to laughing so hard. When I awoke the next morning, the face had rubbed off onto my night-gown. I panicked and called Carol into my room again. 'You have to use an indelible marker this time.' I was determined to show a smiling face to the doctors and nurses. The only comment I received was from one of the nurses, afterward, who told me, 'You certainly are a brave woman.' I don't know about that, but I was determined not to let this cancer get the best of me."

In August 1993, at age forty-four, Claudia Berryman-Shafer thought she noticed a difference in one breast, but ignored it. "Every once in a while, I would feel something, but I wasn't really concerned as I'm one of those it-will-never-happen-to-me people. Still am. In October, our school, in conjunction with our insurance company, put on a health fair. They had never sponsored one before nor have they since. As part of the fair, you could sign up for a mammogram. I was due for one and figured that if there was a lump it would show on the mammogram. I was called back after the initial x-rays for more views. The next set was, in the radiologist's words, 'indeterminate,' and I was told to see my doctor to decide if I needed a biopsy. My doctor definitely felt a lump and made an appointment for me with a surgeon. The surgeon also felt a lump but thought it was a type of benign tumor called a fibroadenoma because it moved around. But he wanted to biopsy it. He said, 'All lumps belong in bottles,' meaning that any unusual lump needs to be removed even if it's benign.

"The biopsy was scheduled for three weeks later, after Christmas break. In the meantime, my husband and I had decided to learn how to snowboard. I broke my wrist doing that, so when I went in for my biopsy, I also had pins put in my wrist to help heal the break. I got a 'two-fer' operation!

"As soon as the surgeon did the biopsy, he knew it was cancer and went out to tell Jim. When I awoke in recovery, my husband was there but the doctor had already left. Jim told me, 'The good news is that your wrist will be fine. The bad news is that you have cancer.'

"I saw the surgeon several days later. He and the oncologist both recommended a mastectomy. The tumor was quite large—three centimeters in diameter—and was classified as Stage 2. As it turned out, the doctors had called it right. When they performed the mastectomy, they found another smaller tumor and cancer cells throughout the breast tissue. A lumpectomy with radiation might have left some cells. Luckily, there was no node involvement, but with Stage 2, chemo is standard protocol."

At the same time that Claudia found out that she had breast cancer, her mother, then seventy-nine, was undergoing chemotherapy for ovarian cancer. "My brother and I agreed that we wouldn't tell Mom about me because it might be too stressful for her. About a month later, Jim and I were getting ready to visit her. I had already started chemo. I thought I should tell her then because my hair was falling out and I knew she'd notice. So I called her and said, 'By the way, I had a mastectomy in January and I recently began chemotherapy.' She said, 'Oh, really?' And then we just sort of finished the conversation. I thought, 'Hmm, that was a strange reaction.'

"She called me the next day and said, 'I was really in shock. I didn't know what to say. Why didn't you tell me before? I would have come to be with you.' I said, 'That's why. You were undergoing your own chemo. You couldn't simply up and leave.' A couple of days later, when we arrived at her house in Southern California, she opened the door and the first thing she said to me was, 'I'm really mad.' So we talked some more. Since then, the whole family has been able to talk about breast cancer and my mom and I have been able to compare experiences, such as, 'So, you're still numb there, too?'"

Nancy Knoble had been visiting her ailing father in the summer of 1993 when she discovered a lump in her breast. "My father had been suffering from a slow-growing form of cancer—carcinoid tumors—for about nine years. Earlier that spring, the tumors had really taken hold and he was failing quickly. I spent that summer going back to Connecticut nearly every weekend to be with my parents. On one visit, I discovered the lump. It was like the one that had been biopsied in 1983, relatively small, hard, distinct. I knew that the chances were great that it was benign. I didn't think it was anything serious. So I waited until after my father had died before I mentioned this to my husband. He urged me to have the lump looked at right away. In fact, he made the appointment for me the next day.

"The doctor basically told me what I already knew: it was a small, hard, detached lump. But it didn't show up in the mammogram. The doctor said, 'I've never seen anything like this be a problem.' I said, 'I'm not comfortable knowing there's a tumor in my body. I want to have it biopsied. I don't want a needle biopsy, either. I don't trust them.' About a week later, on October 8, I underwent a regular surgical biopsy.

"On October 11, the nurse called and said, 'We can't give you these results over the phone. You need to come in.' I went home that evening and said to Dick, 'Guess what, sweetie, I have to go in tomorrow and talk to my doctor about the biopsy results.' He asked, 'What does that mean?' I said, 'Well, she didn't say I had cancer, but I can't imagine—let's think of all the reasons she would want me to come into her office to talk.' We dreamed up a lot of possibilities, but, realistically, I thought I probably had cancer.

"Dick and I went in together the next day and, of course, that was the case. I was lucky. If I had to have cancer, mine was a relatively small invasive tumor, about one centimeter, very clearly Stage 1. I had some DCIS—ductal carcinoma *in situ*—and lobular *in situ* carcinoma. The cancer had broken through the wall of the duct and was starting to invade the rest of the breast tissue. I had a lumpectomy on October 28, 1993."

Thirty-nine-year-old Nancy Johnson also considers herself lucky with her diagnosis. "I had started having annual mammograms when I was thirty-five for two reasons," she states. "I had lumpy, fibrocystic breasts and I had insurance. All my other mammograms had been fine, but this one showed suspicious areas in my left breast. A biopsy revealed cancer in my lobes. I later found out that I also had cancer starting in my right breast that hadn't shown up on the mammogram.

"The technicians were surprised, too, because my last mammogram was only a year old and they claimed that breast cancer doesn't grow this fast. They finally realized that *the new machines* were making the difference. That year, 1990, all accredited clinics had switched over to new, more powerful machines. I guess I was fortunate that 1990 was the year my cancer was diagnosed, because it was very close to spreading into my lymphs.

"I had lobular carcinoma, a rare form that tends to recur in the other breast even if the original cancerous one is removed. This type also doesn't form a lump, so if I had been relying only on self-examination, I wouldn't have found it. That's why I tell women today that it's important to do both self-examination and to have mammograms.

"Most of the cancer was in my chest wall. They gave me the option of removing the left breast and radiating the right breast, or taking both breasts. I didn't like the odds in favor of a recurrence, so I chose to have a bilateral mastectomy.

"As they were wheeling me to the operating room, I kept thinking, 'Maybe I should hold onto that one breast.' As it turned out, I would have had to turn around and go back in. When they biopsied the right breast tissue, they found that the cancer had already started in there, so I felt better about my decision to have both breasts removed.

"I underwent an eight-hour surgery and a long recovery, but I'm glad I got it all done at once," Nancy adds. "Luckily, there was no involvement in my lymph nodes, so I didn't go through chemo or radiation."

Nancy practiced healing visualization and used arnica, an herbal substance, to inhibit pain and inflammation. "My doctor had warned me to expect my scar to look really bruised and bloody at first," she says. "But I took megadoses of arnica before my surgery and the results were incredible. Two days after surgery, Janet and my mom came to be with me while the doctor removed the bandages. 'This might be hard to look at initially,' she said. My scar basically runs from armpit to armpit, but there weren't any bruises at all—a little blood on the bandages, but no bruises. The doctor was shocked and said that she was going to tell all her patients about arnica."

When Claudia Crosetti was diagnosed in 1991, she had not yet met Nancy Johnson. "I went in for a mammogram of my own accord because it was covered by my insurance," says Claudia. "My doctor had told me a couple of years earlier to go in sometime between the ages of thirty-five and forty for a baseline mammogram. When that doctor quit his practice, he recommended a new doctor; the mammogram was sent to him. We weren't following anything, I didn't feel any lumps, there's no history of cancer in my family. I did self-exams, but I had fibrocystic breasts and I wasn't exactly sure what to be looking for and certainly didn't want to find anything. The doctor's office said that they'd call if there was a problem. That's how all my pap tests had been done. They'd call if there was a problem; so I went on my merry way and they never called.

A year later, during her annual physical with the new doctor, a lump was discovered in Claudia's left breast. "He scheduled me for a mammogram," she recounts. "Before the radiologist examined me, he asked, 'Did you have your recommended biopsy last year?' My heart sank to my stomach. I said, 'You mean there is something in my body that should have been taken out a year ago?' I lost it. The doctor said, 'Don't panic. You're young. You'll probably be fine. Don't worry about it.' We scheduled a biopsy right away and took another mammogram.

"Sure enough, there were microcalcifications on the current mammogram and they looked exactly like the ones that had shown up the year before. I asked the doctor, 'Why didn't I get the report? Why didn't anyone tell me about this?' The nurse said, 'Well, maybe it was sent to another doctor whose name also starts with a 'K.'' Nice answer, eh?

"As it turns out, the doctor had no record of it, but the radiologist did. I ended up suing the radiologist and doctor and settling out of court.

"I went to a breast surgeon for the biopsy. She was almost too cool about it. She said repeatedly, 'Don't worry, only twenty percent of women get cancer, you're too young, don't worry about it too much.' I knew absolutely nothing about breast cancer.

"A half hour before I'm to leave work for my follow-up appointment, a *Lear's* magazine article comes across my desk from my boss who'd had a little lump in her breast that had turned out to be nothing. The lump they talked about in the article sounded much like mine. That was the first time it really struck me that I could have cancer. I drove myself to the appointment and was sitting in the waiting room when I heard one of the nurses say in a low voice, 'She's here now.' I thought, 'Not a good sign.'

"The doctor took me into an examination room and didn't ask me right away to take off my clothes so she could examine my stitches. Another bad sign. She started to ask me how I was, and I interrupted her. 'Just tell me. What is it?' She said, 'You have cancer.'

"I felt terrible. I was completely in denial. I said, 'You're kidding!' Then she began to blurt out this information, it's infiltrating ductal and this and that, a bunch of stuff that didn't make any sense to me. My head was spinning because I was feeling all this emotional stuff. I was thinking about my life and death and 'You have cancer,' and seeing this big *thing*.

"I asked her, 'Is it malignant?' because that was the only word I knew in the cancer lingo. She said, 'Yes, it is malignant.' And the first thing I thought about was death. I didn't know about the usual blood, liver and bone tests for another week or so. My life flashed before my eyes.

"The doctor was saying, 'This next year is going to be really aggressive. You are going to need more surgeries. You are going to have chemotherapy.' I'm thinking, 'This happens to other people, people who are sick. I feel fine. This isn't happening to me.' I swear to God, I felt as if my spirit had left my body and I was looking down and watching some incredible conversation taking place between two other people."

It took Claudia several weeks to regain her composure. "I was so angry," she says. "Every time I turned on the TV and saw women with cleavage—who are all over the place—I'd get angry and say, 'Damn this society. Why do breasts have to be so important?'"

Since her tumor was located directly beneath her left nipple, a lumpectomy would have involved taking the nipple, too. "My breast would have been so deformed, it would have looked like a pancake," says Claudia. "The doctors recommended a mastectomy. My breasts weren't small and I didn't like the idea of one being a lot larger than the other, which would be flat. But having a mastectomy was still a tough decision. Part of it concerned sexual identity, and part was the idea of dealing with a prosthesis, which seemed like a drag to me. I was pretty active and I wasn't sure what I was going to do about that. I knew I didn't want any foreign material in my body—no silicone, no saline. I found out about the tramflap reconstruction, which involved using my own abdominal tissue to reconstruct the breast. That sounded more appealing.

"I told myself, 'Just have the breast removed and don't worry about it.' But then I wondered, 'Maybe I'm doing this for all the wrong reasons.' And I'd cry. 'Why am I putting myself through this? Why am I hacking myself up just to make a breast? Am I doing this for myself or for my boyfriend?' It was a hard decision for a lot of reasons, but also because it's such a long surgery. I was under the knife for about eight hours."

Claudia first learned all she could about the procedure. "The plastic surgeon takes a felt pen and shows the general surgeon where he would like the scar to go in order to make a nice breast. Then the general surgeon goes to work and stays within those guidelines as much as he can, with his primary goal being to get all the cancer out. That's most important.

"Then the plastic surgeon takes over and spends about five-and-a-half hours removing my rectus muscle from my abdomen and molding part of it into a breast. He showed me a brochure on the procedure, which included a photograph of a woman lying on a surgical table looking completely dissected. All I could envision was this bloody torso being hacked apart. But I decided to do it.

"I had two weeks to donate two pints of autologous blood before the surgery, and also run around taking and collecting all my tests. I really learned the meaning of impending doom, looking ahead to that surgery. I tried to stay fit and keep my iron high so that I would be in good shape to undergo the operation. It's major, and it leaves you almost unable to walk. I started out walking bent in half, because one of my rectus muscles had been removed—drains hanging all over the place. The doctors said that I'd regain my strength, and I did, but it took a long time."

At age twenty-five, Roberta Fama was deemed "too young" by the medical profession to have breast cancer. "I had been kind of doing self-exams. We had been shown how in high school, but I had very lumpy breasts," says Roberta. "Some of the lumps would come and go with my periods. But this new one had stayed through two or three cycles, so when I went for my annual physical at Planned Parenthood I mentioned it. The nurse said, 'Oh, you're too young, but you might want to have it checked out just to make sure.'

"I found a breast clinic, thinking they would be the experts. I didn't have a regular doctor, so I met with the clinic doctor. He examined me and said, 'Don't worry, it's only thickening; you're too young to have cancer.' I told him that I'd like to have a mammogram anyway. I had to insist. He did one and it came back negative.

"Six months later, the thickening had changed into a lump about the size of a quarter. I had read in the meantime that mammograms aren't one hundred percent effective in detecting breast cancer. I went back to the same doctor at the breast clinic and he basically told me that I was a hysterical female and that I had just had a mammogram six months before, so what was I talking about? I explained that I was getting ready to be married, and I wanted to be absolutely sure. So he agreed to examine me.

"As soon as he felt the lump, he suggested that he do a needle biopsy right there in his office, with no anesthetic. My fiancé Dominic was with me. The doctor kept poking me with the needle but couldn't get much of anything out of the lump. He finally decided to use the little bit of fluid that he did get, which came back negative.

"I thought, 'Great, now I can get back to my life.' Dominic and I got married and went on our honeymoon, a month-long trip to the Philippines. Towards the end of the honeymoon, I noticed some dimpling around the lump. I thought, 'Well, it's not cancer because I just had it biopsied.'

"I had another mammogram after we returned from our trip,

on my twenty-seventh birthday. This one also came back with the report, 'No change from previous year.' I knew that couldn't be true; the dimpling alone was a change. My mother-in-law, who is a nurse, recommended another doctor. He looked at the two mammograms and said that the first one was fine. However, he told me, the second was blurred. Perhaps I had moved during the procedure. In any case, the radiologist had rendered an opinion on a fuzzy film. The new doctor ordered what is called a 'zero mammogram,' which involves a more intense x-ray. The radiologist who performed the mammogram said that although he didn't see anything on the film, he wanted to examine me. He said, 'Since you have something suspicious going on, I think you should have the lump surgically biopsied.' I took the film to another radiologist for a second opinion; he said he didn't see anything, either. They were all saying that it was probably just lumpy tissue.

"But I decided to have another surgical biopsy. We were living with my mother-in-law in Long Beach at the time, and she and Dominic were both with me. When I awoke in recovery, the doctor was standing over me. He said, 'You're okay, but we found cancer.' I went numb. Dominic had left to get me some flowers, so his mother had to go find him so that he could call my parents in Sacramento. They got in the car and drove down immediately.

"The doctors recommended a modified radical mastectomy. I asked what a second opinion offered. They said, 'Lumpectomy and radiation.' I chose the most aggressive treatment—the mastectomy—so that I wouldn't have to second-guess myself later on. The mastectomy left me feeling like I had been hit by a truck. But, that wasn't the worst part. I was home from the hospital when the doctor called. I could tell the minute he said his name, it wasn't good news. He told me that they found some lymph node involvement. They had told me if there was no lymph node involvement, I wouldn't have to go through chemotherapy. Now I would have to.

"I dropped the phone, walked outside and screamed, cried. Dominic ran after me. We finally talked to the doctor again, told him that we were planning on starting a family, and how long would we have to wait? He said at least two years. I asked, 'Why so long, when the chemo is only for six months?' The doctor explained, 'It's not so much the chemo as the fact that the first two years is when most cancers come back. And if it comes back, it will eventually get you.' That's what he told me. I thought, 'Great, every year I'm going to have to take tests that me tell me whether I'm going to live or die?' It was incredibly hard to hear, but of course I agreed to the chemotherapy."

Chemotherapy was prescribed for Andrea Martin *before* surgery. "The tumor was growing so fast that several doctors recommended having chemo first, a procedure that was being used in Europe and therefore called the 'European method,'" says Andrea. "The tumor was seven centimeters. I'd had negative mammograms for years before that. By the time a tumor is palpable or shows up on mammography, it's been growing for seven to ten years."

Calcifications had been removed from Andrea's breast three years earlier. "When they did that surgery, we knew there was another area in the breast that was palpable," she says. "But the doctors said that as long as the lump was soft and movable not to worry about it, but to have a mammogram every six months. If I had known then what I know now, I would have said, 'No way, do a biopsy.' But, as Laura Evans said, 'I heard what I wanted to hear.' I went home happy."

Andrea went home to a very busy life. Having migrated from Memphis, Tennessee, to San Francisco in 1969 with the intent of teaching high school-level French, Andrea had found a dearth of teaching opportunities instead. She taught as a substitute while she returned to school to obtain a law degree. She specialized in medical malpractice. "The firm I worked with represented nearly every hospital in the Bay Area," Andrea states. "My clients were doctors and nurses. My work gave me a peek inside the medical profession, which has since served me well."

During this time, she also married. Her husband, Steve, was a mortgage banker. By 1980, Andrea had tired of practicing law. "It was not the search for truth and justice I thought it was going to be," she quips. Soon afterward she opened a Memphis-style barbecue restaurant called Hog Heaven. "It was very successful," she says. "Steve's business was successful. We lived the lifestyle of the eighties, in excess."

Their daughter, Mather, was born in 1982. The marriage unraveled several years later. In 1986, Andrea sold Hog Heaven and took a breather. "I had met my current husband, Richard, in 1987, and we pursued an idyllic courtship," she recollects. They were married in 1988. During the winter holidays, Richard's sister died of breast cancer at age forty-nine. Two weeks later, Andrea found out that she had breast cancer.

"I was scared out of my life," she says. "I had an aggressive tumor. The look on the doctors' faces when I came in for my results—*wow!* The biopsy showed the cancer was invasive, infiltrating, ductal, Stage 3 plus. It was in my nodes. I had lumps under my arm. They did not expect me to survive; gave me a forty percent chance of living for the next five years. All I could think was, 'I've got this darling little daughter. I have a wonderful husband. I have a great life.' The torment, especially at night, was incredible. I kept asking myself, 'How can I convey to

Mather what I need to before I die? Should I leave her letters to read later?'

"I remember, right before my diagnosis, I had gone into a depression. I had no reason to be depressed. I was in love. It was the holidays. Now, I realize, my body was fighting cancer and getting depressed. I really sunk into it once I began treatment. I had six rounds of chemo, then six weeks of radiation, which really zapped me. After radiation, I would have begged, borrowed or stolen to find one doctor who would tell me that I didn't have to do another eight rounds of chemo. But they said that you have to keep throwing the poison at the cancer cells as they divide, to make sure you get them.

"I thought it made sense to do the chemo before surgery, to address the problem in the most direct way. The cancer had already gone into my nodes, into my lymph system. I wanted to get that 'Drano' in there. I trusted my instincts. If the chemo was going to work, the doctor said, we'd see the tumor recede. And we did."

During the first series of treatments, Andrea's doctor gave her Cytoxan, 5-Fluorouracil and Adriamycin (called CFA). After radiation treatment, he changed the protocol to Cytoxan, Methotrextate and 5-Fluorouracil (called CMF), to avoid damage to Andrea's heart from too much Adriamycin.

Andrea will never forget the first time she received her chemo "cocktail." "The doctor took out this huge syringe about as fat as a half dollar, full of red liquid, cold out of the refrigerator. He stood there and slowly injected all of it into my vein, no dripping from an IV. It took about ten minutes to get it all into me. To this day, if I smelled that cocktail, I'd puke."

The doctor also gave Andrea a shot of Compazine, and sent her home with a Compazine suppository, to help fight the expected nausea. "He said, 'I'll see you in three weeks,'" Andrea recalls. "Five hours later, I'm sitting in bed, high as a kite, strangely energized by the drugs. I called my father and said, 'Dad, if this is what it's going to be like, it's not that bad. I can do this.' I hung up and tossed my cookies. I threw up every minute for the next eight hours. When I had nothing left inside, I retched. Two days later, my hair started falling out. It was gone in two weeks. I've never had a period after that first treatment. I was forty-two."

After her first round of chemotherapy, Andrea Martin joined a cancer support group to "find out if this happened to other women," she says. "We started out with fifteen women. By 1995, six years later, only seven were left." This disturbing fact was a significant signpost pointing the way toward the development of the Breast Cancer Fund and its alliance with Expedition Inspiration.

Treatment

THE WOMEN OF EXPEDITION INSPIRATION discovered that the process of diagnosing and treating breast cancer is also a process of education. For these women, and for many others afflicted with the disease, the process can become a journey from a point of innocence and fear to a plateau of wisdom and determination.

As each team member discovered, different stages and types of cancer call for different treatments. There is an arsenal of medical "weapons" available to fight the disease, from surgery, chemotherapy and radiation to bone marrow reconstitution, immunotherapy and hormone-blocking therapy. Many types of alternative medical approaches are also available to help deal with the effects of surgery and treatment. For each woman afflicted with breast cancer, the hardest decision often is whether to have a lumpectomy or mastectomy—when that choice is allowed.

Laura, Nancy Knoble, Annette and Kim elected to have lumpectomies. The others chose, or were prescribed, mastectomies.

Andrea Martin underwent a mastectomy after two months of chemotherapy that had shrunk the tumor to half its original size. "The surgery was the easy part, compared to chemotherapy," she says. "I had three more rounds of Adriamycin after surgery. That was a struggle."

She sought alternative healing methods to help her through the treatment. "I went to a holistic healing center in the California desert, started taking homeopathic remedies to help control nausea and keep my energy level up, used colors for meditation, tried prayer, acupuncture and herbs," she says. "I put as much in my arsenal as I could, including aravan, which I learned about in my support group. Aravan helped me sleep right after the infusions. I never threw up after the second round of chemo. I also shaved my head to avoid having to watch my hair fall out."

The accumulative effects of chemotherapy often play havoc with the brain, temporarily scrambling short- and long-term memory. "It's called 'chemo-brain,'" says Andrea, "and it takes quite awhile to regain your full mental capacity, once chemo has ended."

But end it did, and Andrea got on with her life by joining Dianne Feinstein's 1990 campaign for governor of California. "I felt an urgent need to have women in high-level offices helping to make decisions that affect women's lives," says Andrea. After Feinstein lost the election, Andrea was appointed the Northern California Deputy Finance Director for Feinstein's bid for the U.S. Senate. "Just as we were starting a huge fundraising campaign, I found a lump in my remaining breast. I was leaning over, brushing my teeth and doing a routine breast check with my free hand. I felt a hard, pebble-like lump that I had never felt before."

Andrea waited two weeks to see if the lump would disappear; it didn't. Her surgeon performed a biopsy. "As soon as he cut into it, he knew it was cancer," she says.

That was in 1991, about a year after she had finished her last chemo, two years after her first diagnosis. Fortunately, this was not a metastasis but rather a new, primary site, less than one centimeter and non-aggressive. The doctor advised a lumpectomy with no chemo, no radiation. Andrea told him, "No, thank you, I'm having a mastectomy. Take it off. At least I'll be symmetrical again."

She and Richard left the surgeon's office high-fiving. "If you have to have breast cancer, this is what you want," she explains. "I conducted a successful kickoff fundraiser for Dianne on Thursday night, had the mastectomy on Friday and was back to work in two weeks. I began taking Tamoxifen, a powerful drug that is supposed to help prevent recurrences."

Everything Kim had read about lumpectomies versus mastectomies showed that the cure rate was about the same. "It was a borderline decision because of the size of the mass," she says. "They didn't know how much of the breast they could conserve because they took out a mass about the size of a tennis ball. I had axillary node dissection and no node involvement, which was really good news. The doctors had prepared me to expect node involvement because of the large size of the tumor."

Kim was in denial right up to the morning of her surgery. "We took Evan to the hospital with us and I breast-fed him, thinking that maybe when they got in there, they'd find that it really wasn't breast cancer," she says. "Evan was six months old."

Doctors found mostly interductal cancer and some invasive that had spread from one duct to another. "It was estrogen receptive," says Kim, "meaning that it might have hastened the growth of the cancer. I was one of the few lactating women the doctors had ever performed a lumpectomy on. That was a challenge—having to deal with my breast milk drying up as well as the surgery. Drying up was more painful than surgery. Both breasts became inflamed and I had to use ice packs on them. Eventually because of the surgery, chemicals and anesthesia, both breasts stopped producing milk altogether. I was treated with radiation for seven weeks and then chemotherapy for six months."

The doctor recommended a special Canadian protocol that substituted Leukovorin for Cytoxan. Cytoxan can sometimes destroy ovaries and Art and Kim thought they might have more children.

Like many of the team members, Kim has always been physically active and fit, and found this to be a boon to her recovery. "I tried to continue to run during the whole ordeal," she says. "I hadn't run during the final months of my pregnancy, but I started back up when Evan was five weeks old. It really helped me feel better. I knew I could get the toxins out of my body a lot faster, so I'd do chemo on Friday and run on Saturday. Initially, I didn't feel so great, but by evening, I could tell that running a 5K had helped."

Kim struggled to maintain a normal routine for Evan's first year. She returned to work when Evan was about a year old. She had chemotherapy on Fridays, leaving Saturday and Sunday to recuperate when Art was home. They also moved to a new house during this time.

"I couldn't have made it without Art and my mom and dad," Kim says. "Mom drove to our house every day, an hour each way, to care for Evan. After my surgery, I couldn't lift the baby for six weeks. I had a Jackson-Pratt drain pump that went in through my rib cage. Mom weaned Evan onto a bottle while I was in the hospital. I realized that people who have a supportive family are very fortunate. I always think about how difficult it must be for people who don't have that support."

Although raised a Roman Catholic, over the years Kim had become more eclectic about religion and spirituality. "For me, having cancer never caused a questioning of faith. I knew that God had given me the power to make decisions, the power to fight the cancer, as well as free will and a positive mental attitude. There was also a feeling of letting go of control, of knowing that having cancer was out of my hands and that I'd make the best of it. In some ways, it was a great relief, and it was also a gift. You realize that it doesn't do any good to worry about what might happen. You have to appreciate the moment and beauty of everything. I know my friends got kind of fed up with me talking about the beauty of the sunrise, the trees, the flowers, but I see things through an artist's eyes anyway. Everything had become more enhanced.

"Things that used to bother me don't bother me as much anymore—being late, being on time, being a perfectionist. In the past, if I got hung up in traffic and thought I'd be late for an appointment, I'd be a wreck. By realizing how focused I was on being perfect, I found out how far from perfect I am. It was a release to become more comfortable with myself, more appreciative of myself.

"When you're diagnosed with cancer, you go through a grieving process—not at the level of mourning the death of a family member or friend, but there is a grieving. It's important to take the time to experience this. I saw it as both grieving and celebrating, the closure of one episode of my life and the opening of a whole new chapter. One woman I know refers to her life as 'B.C. and A.D.—Before Cancer and After Diagnosis.' That's a good way to explain the significant change that occurs, the loss of innocence.

"I know that our society has come a long way in helping people deal with going through life-threatening illnesses, but we still have a long way to go in terms of offering support to families, spouses and partners. At times, Art was extremely supportive and helpful. Other times, he didn't have the emotional strength to help me or Evan because he was so focused on how badly he was feeling."

After her surgery, Ashley focused on her feelings of anger. "It was too scary," she remembers. "The whole first year after my surgery, I volunteered at the American Cancer Society and went to other groups for support, but many of them were for other cancers or young kids with leukemia. I couldn't find any groups with young girls with breast cancer. I told the doctor, 'I want people my age. Find me another teenager who has breast cancer.' But he couldn't. I got very depressed and sad and I cried a lot. Each January, the anniversary month of my mastectomy, I'd get really depressed and cry all the time."

Before her surgery, Ashley had enjoyed an active social life. "Afterward," she says, "I found I couldn't do it anymore. I remember the first time I went to a bar to hang out with my buddies and listen to some jazz, sing a couple of tunes, and the first time I had one vodka tonic—I just got trashed. I used to be able to put down six or seven. I mean, I partied *very* hard in high school. People whale on me now because I don't go out and party with them anymore. They're all my age. I'm thinking, 'Been there, done that.'"

Ashley adds, "I remember lying in the hospital bed after my mastectomy. It's about two in the morning and I'm channel surfing. And there are pictures of Kuwait, and how they bombed the hell out of it. I'm watching this and I'm already all emotional and I'm thinking all these people in Kuwait are being killed and maimed and harmed for no reason. I didn't understand Saddam Hussein. I thought if he were lying here in a hospital bed with testicular cancer, he'd have a different view on this. It totally blew my mind why somebody would want to inflict pain on other people when there are already so many people suffering already. The whole experience came down to one thought: I don't understand the need to cause human suffering.

"I grew up with religion, but it didn't become part of my life. I wish it had, though. When the doctor came in after my mastectomy, he told me that they had found more cancer, and then he left. I was lying there with the news when my mom's friend, Billie Doyle, came in to visit me. She brought me flowers. At the time, she had been dealing with breast cancer for two years—she died a few years later—and she happened to be there when I found out. It was a good sign, I think, because she was a very spiritual woman, very religious, like my mom. The two of them could look at cancer and dying with a strong degree of faith. That was the one thing I was missing. I didn't have a belief in God. I always felt very empty, as if there was no point to it all. I figured, just go with the flow, deal with what you've been given.

"Now I strive to be like my mother. I've been more caring and I try to be a good person. That's as close as I can get to a feeling of spirituality. But there are days when I feel like snapping at people and being a rude bitch. I just keep checking myself."

≈

Sara could have had a lumpectomy, as she explained. "The statistics on the East and West Coasts were leaning towards lumpectomies. But here in the Midwest, we're very conservative and still doing mostly mastectomies. I deferred to Fritz and my surgeon. The surgeon cleaned me out—took the breast and twenty-two lymph nodes. Luckily, I didn't have to have radiation or chemotherapy because my nodes were negative.

"I remember the anesthesiologist calling me at home the night before my surgery. He said, 'Mrs. Hildebrand, I'm Dr. So-and-so and I'll be doing your anesthesia tomorrow.' I said, 'Fine.' He said, 'Tell me, do you get to the mall very often?' And I thought, this guy's going to assess my physical condition on that question? Here in Wisconsin, when the weather is bad, everyone goes to the mall to walk for exercise. I prefer to run outside. But I said, 'Sure, I *can*.' And he said, 'Okay, then, I'll see you tomorrow.' And that was it. Later, when I decided to apply for the team, I remember thinking, 'Should I walk around the mall for the rest of my life or should I go to the mountain?'

"Fritz helped me through it all for the first two weeks between the diagnosis and the surgery. I had the surgery on a Tuesday and finished the pain pills about four days later and thought, 'Boy, I like these pills.' But the surgeon said, 'No more, you're finished.' Then the reality dawned on me that I really had breast cancer and it scared me. I read all sorts of books and then I wasn't sleeping well at night. I told myself, don't read anything after dinner about breast cancer, or, better yet, stop reading. You've learned everything there is to learn, there are no answers."

Still, the question of how she got breast cancer continued to haunt Sara. "After I got home from the hospital, I moped around, trying to figure it out. I could not lift my arm to the top of my head for three months. The gal who does my hair did it for free for two months, as a gift to cheer me up. I finally called a good friend and classmate from Smith College, who now lives in New York City. She had had a mastectomy twenty-eight years before and lost her husband over it, but was happily remarried. I said to her, 'You have to help me through this. People around here aren't talking about it. It's too conservative a community. I need some help.' My friend buys and sells corporate art, but also volunteers her time at hospitals, visiting mastectomy patients. If you were to see this gorgeous creature walk in your hospital room you would think, 'Okay, I'm also going to get out of this bed and I will be all right.'

"The first thing she said to me was, 'You have cancer but shortly you will have *had* cancer. It will be a closed book and you will put it in the past.' She called me all the time to reinforce this thought and really helped me a lot."

Eleanor, who originally thought that she did not need support through her illness and treatment, found herself in an emotional nosedive after ending a year of chemotherapy. "The treatment also had plunged me into premature menopause," she says. "My mood changed. I was bothered by my body image and lack of self-worth. I had a lot of anger. I came face-to-face with the fact that 'Hey, Eleanor, there's nobody in charge of this but you.' It upset me because I always felt that I was only appreciated as long as I could do things for other people and not because of just being me. I had to get over that and appreciate myself. A lot of growth came out of the experience, but it was a terrible ordeal. At the same time, my oldest son was entering his teenage years and our family life was just off the wall.

"I don't know whether the chemotherapy got rid of the anger or if it was self-realization or therapy. All I know is that afterward I was a much happier person, which could only have made life better for my family. When you have cancer, you tend to get rid of a lot of baggage. You really have to reorder the way you think. How can you fight about stupid little things such as having to pick up your clothes, or 'Sister said something mean to me'? You can't waste time on this stuff. For me, the cancer began the process of a lot of self-discovery."

On the day of her mastectomy, Patty contemplated the importance of her breasts, with characteristic good humor. She wrote in her journal: "It was time to say good-bye to my boob. Boobs become fond members of the body. They bring you into womanhood and you use them to make yourself attractive. Clothes are designed around boobs and now old 'Itzy' was going to Boob Heaven, leaving 'Bitzy' behind to face T-shirts alone."

After surgery, Patty awoke in a private room with her mother sitting beside the bed. "She took me home and took care of me," says Patty. "We watched movies, and friends and family visited and brought food. Peter would call from Steamboat Springs in distress, wondering what to fix himself and the kids for dinner. I had to remind him to broil the steak, bake the chicken; he'd get it backwards. He did amazingly well taking care of the business, the kids, the dog and the house, and gained a new appreciation for the role of Mom.

"During the mastectomy, the doctors didn't remove any lymph nodes because tubular cancer doesn't spread. A week after the surgery, I saw Dr. Milch with my sister Franny. He said not only did I have tubular cancer but I also had ductal and lobular, so could he take a look at my lymph nodes—how about the day after tomorrow?"

Cancer suddenly became more real, more life-threatening to Patty, and she broke down. "I sobbed. I was glad my sister was there. She helped me break the news to everyone else."

The next day, Patty started worrying about Christmas, only a few weeks away. She insisted that her sister take her shopping. "With my drain bottle hanging under my armpit, we went shopping. We shopped all day right up to my two o'clock operation. I wasn't allowed to eat or drink anything, and we kept passing these fresh cookie shops. Franny had to drag me away from them."

On December 3, Patty's lymph nodes were removed. "This recovery was not quite the same," she remembers. "Lymph node removal hurts more, limits more movement and leaves more numbness. It was interesting to have had the surgeries done separately and to compare them.

"I was moved to another room, next to a dying woman who had been there for months, with no visitors. She was out of it and I began to wonder if I was here for the same reason. I begged to get out of the hospital early and did, with visiting nurses and Mom caring for me. A new drain was put in place and chemotherapy was just around the corner."

A few days later, a bone scan was performed to check for more cancer. It was negative, but the doctor deemed chemotherapy to be necessary, in case some of the cancer had skipped over the lymph nodes and gone into other organs. Patty had her first dose in Buffalo. "It was the usual mix—Cytoxan, Methotrexate and 5 Fluorourocil (CMF)—plus Prednisone to ease the effect of the chemo. I was afraid of the first shot," Patty says. "Dr. Cooper said that I would not lose my hair; it would just thin out. He said that I would also gain about ten pounds.

"As it turned out, the first shot wasn't that bad. It only took about fifteen minutes to administer. The fluid felt cold as it entered my veins, and left a bad taste in my mouth, which explains the candy dishes in the treatment room. I was put on a schedule to receive chemo every week for three months, then every two weeks for another three months. As the drugs built up in my system, I started feeling bad. I found that I had to take this feeling and set it to the side, like paperwork on my desk. It was still there but it could be displaced. Each person finds a way of dealing with this feeling, from meditation to marathon running."

After her first chemo shot, Patty decided to talk to her oldest sister, Sally, who was having a rough time with alcohol. "I told her, 'If I can put this shit in my body to get better, you can take that shit out of your body and get better. It's hurting you on the inside exactly like the cancer is hurting me. I want my sister back and I don't have her when she's drinking.' I figured, if I'm going to die, I might as well tell her what I think. By the next summer, she had quit drinking and hasn't had a drink since. I have my sister back and she's better than ever."

Patty made it home in time for Christmas with her boys and the dog. There were presents under the tree and full stockings hanging from the mantle. Although she was anxious to get back to a normal routine, Patty was continually besieged with severe side effects from the chemo, including mouth sores, hemorrhoids, bleeding fissures and abdominal pain. "The pain was the worst for four or five days following chemotherapy," she recollects. "The second three-month chemo schedule called for a dose every two weeks. In the beginning, the second week was a blessing, a time when I felt a little better, but after a month it was bad all the time. I called Dr. Cooper and begged to quit early. No chance. After my shot, I would drive home and curl up in bed from the abdominal pain. I never threw up. The overall nauseous feeling never went away; it just hit different levels. The best medicine was to keep busy, be active. I skied during the winter, worked in our retail store, helped my son's school raise money, decorated for a cabaret show and went on long walks with our

Labrador retriever, Ewik. Having a faithful dog to share your time is always good. She would run or walk beside me and be happy, or curl up beside me when I'd have to lie down.

"The drugs made my stomach bloat out as if I were five months pregnant. My face looked puffy and round, my hair thin. I definitely looked different, but I was alive and chemo was almost over. It took some time—over a month—to feel better after my last shot. But at last I could eat healthfully and get back in shape."

Since Vicki was the main source of financial support for herself and her children, she tried to schedule everything around her job. "I scheduled surgery for November 18 so I could recuperate over the Thanksgiving holiday," she says. "Larry went with me. I didn't want to be tranquilized, but finally let them give me a little before they wheeled me down the hall into the operating room. I kept thinking that someone might come bursting in, saying, 'We goofed! Those were someone else's tests.' I wouldn't let them put me under until I saw my doctor.

"I had my hand on my breast going in there, and when I woke up, my hand was still there but my breast wasn't. The next day, my doctor came in to take off my bandages. Both Larry and Joyce, a good friend from Portland, were there. I said, 'I hope you guys don't mind if I don't look.' I had my head back as far as I could stretch. The doctor said, 'That's fine, take your time. You don't need to look at this.' Of course, right away, I'm asking Joyce and Larry, 'What does it look like? What is he doing?' So they gave me a blow-by-blow. Larry said, 'It's not so bad looking.' That was the last time Larry ever looked at my scar willingly.

"Later that afternoon, after Larry had left and only Joyce and I were in the room, I told her, 'I want out of my hospital gown and I want my real clothes on and I want to see it.' I stood in front of the mirror and looked. There were small bandages over the incision, and I was surprised that it really didn't look so bad. The area was swollen, so it looked kind of nubile. When I got home, I showed it to any of my women friends or family who wanted to see it. My father never did want to look at it, but Mom did."

Vicki's chemo treatments started right after Thanksgiving. "The last few months of chemo were hard because chronic illness gets tiring for people," she explains. "Friends, as wonderful and dear as they are, have to get back to their lives. Surgery is a black-and-white thing. You have it, it's over. But chemo goes on and on. It took its toll on Larry. He started to fade and my kids started taking on more responsibility the last couple of months. I was really sick then. I don't know what I would have done without Katy and Jonathan."

Nancy Hudson's two young boys also were a comfort to her. "David caught me crying in my room one night when I was recovering from the mastectomy. I also had my leg propped up because of a knee injury," she says. "I was watching Bill Moyers's program on healing with the mind. The program struck a chord in me and I burst out crying. I'm normally very active, so here are my boys, watching me hobble around and cry. David came in and started crying, too, then Nick joined us. They couldn't stand to see me cry.

"I told them it was okay, it was good that we were crying and that this was a really tough time. Their dad already had moved out, then I got breast cancer, and I hurt my knee—I realized how scary this must be for them. They said, 'Mom, turn off this program. Let's watch something else.' Good idea. Time to switch programs."

Sue Anne began to concentrate on developing her own program of treatment and recovery. A doctor she consulted advised her to take the strongest dose of chemo she could get. "I had three months of Adriamycin and five months of CMF," says Sue Anne. "They also gave me antinausea pills. I was totally whacked out for a week after the first round. It hit the second day. I took the antinausea pills the first time because I wanted to be a good patient. The next round, I didn't take them at all and I felt much better.

"Each of those first three sessions was like being dead. I had no energy. After I finished chemo, they sent me for six weeks of radiation, five days a week. That wasn't all that terrible. I didn't get as tired; it was just a hassle to go every day. I continued to teach my class in creativity at the local college. I formed my own support network. I met with a group of nurses and relied on many friends. I feel as if it took an army of friends to get me through this.

"My children were in school during the whole ordeal. They had to fend for themselves. My husband by then had isolated himself in one corner of the house and we were not communicating. Our household was disintegrating around us and it was hard on the kids, but they managed."

Sue Anne's oldest daughter, Mignon, composed an essay about her mother's cancer experience:

"My mom and I have our tough times, like probably most moms and daughters," Mignon wrote when she was thirteen. "But in 1992, things got even tougher, when she was diagnosed with breast cancer. Sometimes I felt as if I was her parent. I had to fill in when she couldn't do the usual things around the house. There were more chores and less special time for me.

"It's hard not to get swallowed up in fear just hearing the word *cancer*. You can't help but wonder just how long she'll be around for you. When her hair started to fall out because of the chemotherapy treatments, she tried to keep her sense of humor by letting my sister and me shave her hair into a Mohawk. Everybody at school knew my mom had cancer. The kids were curious when they saw my mom take her wig off, trying not to be self-conscious and letting them see she was still my mom.

"One way she tried to keep positive during those days without hair was to imagine that she was a Buddhist nun rather than a person with cancer. My mom and I once met a very interesting Buddhist nun (they shave their heads) when we walked with her cross-country in honor of Native Americans. This woman walked tall and proud and I think she was a kind of role model for my mom.

"My mom worked hard to deal with her feelings about our struggle with cancer. She is an art therapist and she really believes in drawing, painting and writing in a diary to help sort out thoughts and feelings. It seems unfair when something like cancer or another tragedy strikes a family. But for us the cancer has brought us closer together. It has taught us to slow down and look at each day and each challenge."

But Sue Anne was struggling with each step. "Cancer was an adjunct to what was going on in my life; the depression, the disintegration of my relationship and my sense of self," she says. "Before my cancer, in my desperation, I had arranged chairs in a circle in the kitchen and called to all wise souls, souls I had known who had gone before, my mother who had died in 1978. I cried, 'I give up. I've tried all my psychological tricks, all my friends' therapists, everything, and I can't do this. I need help.'

"When my mother died, I had this image of a whole group of people she had known in a circle on the ceiling of her bedroom, swooping her up. I trust these communiqués because they are the only consistency I know in my deepest being. All the time I was depressed, I was asking for dreams because they have been my vehicle for guidance. During my depression, I wondered, 'Why am I not getting dreams?' I think a part of me was locked up too tightly."

Sue Anne had never feared death. "I love being alive," she says, "yet I'm not afraid of the transition out of my body. I've always said that I expect death to be a beautiful, 'breathtaking' adventure! I have always been rather defiant about fitting into statistical predictions. I figure if you engage in life to the fullest, when it's time to go it should be a celebration, not a morbid event."

Annette also developed a unique perspective on cancer survivor statistics. "The doctors were telling me that because lymph nodes were involved, the chance of a recurrence was fifty percent. I finally realized that these statistics are meaningless. Either you get it or you don't. It's either one hundred percent or zero, isn't it?"

Like her teammates, Annette also took a long, hard look at her life during her cancer experience. "To me, the process was like making reduction sauce. You just boil it and boil it and boil it until all you're left with is the absolute essence. I don't think I'm a different person since cancer, but what wasn't me has boiled away."

During her chemotherapy, Annette practiced visual imagery. "I used it for healing. Every time I got chemo, I'd do a visualization tape, to aid the chemicals in doing their job and to help control my fear. For years, I had watched my diet; no white bread, low fat, lots of salads, limited red meat. So the thought of putting this stuff in my body—you know, the nurses are pulling on rubber gloves because you can't let the chemo drugs touch your skin because they would eat the skin away. But somehow they're okay in your veins? And I'm going to get my lifetime dosage of Adriamycin in one fell swoop and if you get too much of that it could blow out your heart? I needed the visualization to help me control the fear that what I was doing was totally irrational."

Annette's chemotherapy involved an aggressive protocol that shortened the overall duration of the treatment but increased the dosage. She received chemo every three weeks for four months, followed by five weeks of daily radiation treatment.

"The worst side effect I experienced was to lose my vision for three days after each chemo dose," Annette says. "The first time it happened, with my fear of the chemo anyway, I thought, 'Oh great. Now I'm going to go blind, too!' I always received the dose on a Friday, so that I could recuperate over the weekend. I could see well enough to get around my house, but I couldn't see well enough to read or watch television. There were no distractions. I was left totally alone with myself."

Annette describes her treatment as a powerful experience. "It turned out to be a microcosm of my whole family experience. I grew up in a family that didn't know how to be there for each other. We're nice to each other, but nobody shows up. I grew up in Venezuela, where my father worked for an international paper company. I went away to boarding school in Massachusetts when I was fourteen. My parents never came to see me. And they weren't with me when I went through cancer. I had asked my mother to accompany me to M.D. Anderson, when I was first going around to get opinions, but she felt as if she couldn't do it. One brother came to see me during my treatments, the other didn't.

"I had a lot of time to sort through these feelings during my treatment. I took the opportunity to look at this dysfunction as an adult and to undo some of the anger. I was fortunate to be in group therapy. I ended up coming to a place of accepting that things are not going to change. The challenge for me was, 'So what are you going to do about it?' I finally realized that looking at my family was less horrifying than looking at cancer. And that led me to a whole new playing field, a whole new end to the scale of horrifying possibilities.

"I also came to the realization that it made sense that the cancer had manifested itself as breast cancer on my right side, the feminine, intuitive side. I grew up in a male-dominated family. I was always trying to meet my parents' expectations and, at the same time, was rebelling against them. I got into a job that didn't really express my nature, a linear, analytical job which I was good at, but all the time I was repressing the feminine, creative side of myself. That's why the cancer became such a wake-up call. I had to stop this behavior before I killed myself!

"Having breast cancer helped reinforce my spirituality. It helped me deal with fear, with the need to control; it helped me release anger. It also helped me incorporate the reality of death into life and to appreciate life as a gift. I learned if you give out love you get tons back. And you can keep giving it out because the love doesn't come from a place that empties out; it's continually replenished."

During this time, Annette also learned about miracles. "There were big and little miracles," she says. "People would show up with exactly the right thing at the right time—a reassuring phrase, an act of kindness from somebody I didn't even know. I became very close to my next-door neighbor, who was pregnant. We decided that there were actually a lot of similarities between chemotherapy and pregnancy. We both were exhausted all the time. We both started forgetting everything. We slept a lot, puked a lot, peed a lot. We both rode an emotional roller coaster. At the end of it, she had a baby and I felt reborn."

Mary had more than enough family support to see her through what turned out to be a record short hospital stay. "When I told my doctor that I wanted to leave the morning after my surgery, he said, 'We've never sent anyone home in twenty-four hours.' I told him, 'I want to get out of here. I've got to get hiking again.' I also asked, 'When you do the surgery, be careful of my pectoral muscles. I've spent a lot of time building them up and I need them for my hiking and biking.' I really badgered him. After my surgery, he sent in his assistant to insert a drain in my breast. He showed me how to use it to make sure that the wound drained properly, and said I could go home. The woman in the other hospital bed said, 'Are you sure you just had a mastectomy?'"

Mary's family gathered at the hospital to escort her home. "They had balloons and all the grandkids were there. It was wonderful."

On Monday, Mary's daughter took her shopping. "I was a little woozy, but I didn't let it bother me," says Mary. "My sister came to visit me on Tuesday and we walked up Bradbury Mountain, a little hill nearby, to look at the view."

Throughout the whole ordeal, Bill was quietly supportive. "My husband is not a vocal person," says Mary. "I could feel his support though, and he was wonderful about it. I could tell he was grimacing with me every time I moved my arm. But I was bound and determined to keep that arm strong. Once he said to me, 'Stand up straight, be proud and go on with your life. You're as good as anyone, as good as you ever were.' That was a lot for him to say, and it meant a lot to me."

Mary returned to work at L.L. Bean at the end of November, after climbing nearby 4,000-foot Carter Dome with her sons, Michael and Bill, Jr. "It was six weeks after my surgery," she recalls. "We were in full winter mountain gear. My sons led me up there, took care of me, made sure I was okay. It was a wonderful outing.

"I've always gone into each day with quite a bit of enthusiasm, but not with the intensity that I do now," Mary adds. "Before cancer, I thought I had forever to live. But now, I look at a day differently and try to get everything I can out of it. I try to learn something new, do something new, see something new. And I take it one day at a time, because I don't know how many of these days I have left."

Since Claudia Berryman-Shafer's mother had survived breast cancer for thirty years, Claudia also entered her chemo treatment with a perspective of survival. "The hardest part for me was how the chemotherapy would affect my activities," she says. "I had all these races planned. I decided to go ahead and run them. I finished all of them, although farther back in the pack than I'm used to.

"I rarely get sick. Even as a kid, some bug would go through the whole school system and there I'd be, all alone at school, not sick. As I got older and began to think that illness was mostly stress related, I also thought, 'I must be dealing with my stress in a good way'—until I got cancer. Then it was like, 'Whoa, this must be something that just happened to me'—not related to stress, of course.

"As I got farther away from the effects of the chemo, I started to look back at what had been going on in my life and realized that there had been some pretty heavy stresses. I had taken on the job of teaching the alternative classroom, where all the underprivileged problem kids were sent. In the classroom, I saw a lot of progress, but outside the classroom, where there was no reinforcement, there was no progress. They were still problem kids and still getting into trouble. Everyone expected some sort of miracle cure for everything that was wrong with these kids. I got to where I wouldn't even go to the lunchroom because I'd hear all these pointed comments about 'my kids.' That was real stressful. And I deal with stress by not reacting. I never made any comments back to the other teachers.

"Also, at that same time, my mom was ill. We were told that she'd live a year and I think I was preparing myself for that. But it wasn't something I'd talk about. I just dealt with it internally.

"Jim and I also had a problem selling one house and moving to another. The old house ended up not selling and we had to overlap mortgage payments for a while. That was a strain, with both of us on teachers' salaries.

"All these things added up to more stress than I was aware of. I asked myself what I might be getting out of being sick. I know it got me out of a stressful situation at school. 'Oh, my gosh, she has cancer, so now we can't give her a bad time.' People stopped making remarks, which lifted a big burden. And I went back to teaching sixth grade instead of the alternative class. My mom's illness was resolved—she's already outlived her prognosis by several years—which was a great relief. I made it a point to take time every day to see what stresses might be present and what I could do about them."

Nancy Knoble's breast cancer was only one of many stresses that seemed to happen all at once. "In January, Dick lost his job.

In June, we moved into a new house. In July, my father died. In September, we started renovating the house: gutted the whole thing, put in a new foundation, a new roof, new heating, while we lived in one room downstairs. In October, I was diagnosed with breast cancer. It was almost the least of my problems at the time," says Nancy. "It was a very emotional time for us. It took me a long time to get over my father's death. Dick had been very much a part of that. He spent most of that summer with my dad, with me flying back to join them every weekend.

"Then, right after I had my lumpectomy, I started radiation. Based on the pathology from the lumpectomy, I was encouraged to have radiation only, no chemotherapy. I had radiation five days a week for seven weeks. I'd go in for my treatment in the afternoon, then go home. I commuted an hour each way to work, which made for a long day anyway. I felt as if I had the flu all the time. I was exhausted. By eight o'clock at night, I'd be falling asleep no matter where I was. What surprised me, although I had been told otherwise but refused to believe it, was that when I stopped radiation the effect didn't go away the next day. I expected to be full of energy within a week or two. The reality was, it took two or three months before I got my energy back.

"I tried to stay active and maintain a level of fitness. But, I am not a good regular workout person. I go in spurts. I'd be wonderful for a week or two, then terrible for a week or two. It's amazing that I've been able to run marathons and climb mountains with the kind of sporadic workout schedule I have. I'm erratic. I'm really a weekend warrior."

Although Nancy Johnson was very fit from leading an active, healthy lifestyle, it took her nearly a year to fully recuperate from her bilateral mastectomy. "I had a lot of pain that was difficult to deal with," she says. "I was used to being active and I had to realize that my activity was going to be restricted for a while. I was on morphine right after the surgery, then on other pain medication for about three months. I had been using visualization for various things for years, and used it all through the cancer ordeal. Prior to surgery, I visualized myself healthy. I visualized no cancer in my lymph nodes. One particular visualization I use involves angels. I see little angels flying around inside my body and their faces are people I know. If I feel hot and feverish, the angels pour buckets of cool water on the inside of my body. If I feel pain, they rub it away. This has always worked well for me. I've believed in angels since I was a little girl."

Claudia Crosetti's recuperation also was lengthy, although when she first awoke from surgery, she felt euphoric. "Another woman who'd had the tramflap operation had warned me that I would feel as if I'd been run over by a truck," says Claudia. "I was so riddled with morphine, I felt great at first. But I was completely disoriented. For a couple of days, I went between high and low, feeling really good and having very dark hallucinations. I was on a respirator for a while and I hated that, the idea of something helping me to breathe. I didn't like being hooked up to all this stuff and I'd get anxiety attacks."

Claudia was in the hospital in San Francisco in August 1991, for a week. "I had surgery on August 19. I'll never forget that date because that's the same date that Gorbachev was ousted from power in the Soviet Union," she says. "At least I had something to watch on TV."

Her mother and father rented a small apartment nearby to be with Claudia. "My dad played solitaire, watched a little TV with me when I wasn't sleeping. When I went home, my mom came and stayed with me for two weeks, which was wonderful.

"One of the best things to come out of all this was my relationship with my father. He took me to most of my doctor appointments because I had to travel to San Francisco and needed somebody with me. My mother was really devastated when she first heard the news. She fell apart. My father was pretty calm and he started educating himself about breast cancer. So that gave me somebody to talk to about everything. He was always there for me. He knew I lived alone and told me to call him anytime. I learned a lot about him on those trips to San Francisco. I'm sure it had to do with looking at my own mortality and thinking, 'I'm not taking anyone for granted anymore.' We became close. I have three sisters and we had a good childhood, but a lot of our attention was group attention. This was one of the few times that my dad and I had some time alone."

Because two of fourteen of Claudia's lymph nodes tested positive, the cancer was classified as Stage 2 and chemotherapy was prescribed. "Even though the cancer hadn't shown up in my bone, blood and liver tests, they believed that some cells could be floating around out there," Claudia explains. "They gave me chemo to kill off any stray cancer cells."

Claudia started chemo in September. "I'd go to Dr. Grant once a month in San Francisco, then go to a doctor in Ukiah under her prescription. My white blood cell count was really low, so during the last two months of chemo I had to give myself Neupogen shots, to bolster my count. They can't give you chemo if your count is below a certain number, and mine kept falling, so Dr. Grant finally changed the protocol to include Neupogen. It took me about twenty minutes the first time, to work up the nerve to give myself a shot. After that, it was okay. I didn't like the ritual, though, of 'shooting up.' But I did it. Now, I figure, it's part of my war story."

Every time she had an appointment with Dr. Grant, Claudia asked about her prognosis. "I'd ask a lot of questions, but the bottom line was, 'Am I going to live?' Dr. Grant would say, 'I think your prognosis is pretty good, eighty percent chance, blah, blah, blah.' She never got impatient with my asking those questions. I liked Dr. Grant. I liked being treated by a woman. One of the first things she advised me was, 'Don't make any major changes in your life this year.'

"She asked me if I had a hobby. I took that as a signal and I started taking guitar lessons and playing the guitar very badly. I had taken classical lessons when I was a kid. It became a daily ritual for me, a complete distraction from my cancer preoccupation. Chemo sort of controls your life. I found solace in playing the guitar.

"At the beginning, I didn't know if my cancer was fatal or not. My life had flashed before me when I first received my diagnosis and it happened again a few other times and made me feel very lonely. The simplest things would happen, such as when I was in the Sierra Nevada Mountains in a lodge and there was this old, nostalgic music playing and all these young people having a good time. I felt like this lonely person who was dying. Even after I found out that the cancer hadn't metastasized, there were times when I was just really scared. It was the first time I looked at my mortality, and it was hard. There were some very depressing days. And then there was a gift to it, too. It made me live my life more fully."

Claudia countered her fear and intermittent depression in several ways. "I cut my work schedule down to a five-hour day. I'd walk at least two miles a day. I'd soak in the tub every night, and write in my journal. Journal writing helped me work through some of my emotions. I'm single; I live alone with my cat. All these rituals helped me get through chemo and the fear."

Other than her father, mother and sisters, Claudia didn't have a support group. "There was a support group for cancer in our town, but not one for breast cancer," she recalls. "I went to one group and it was a little too depressing for me. There were people dying of brain tumors. When I started taking Tamoxifen, I had a really terrible time with hot flashes and somebody recommended that I try Tai Chi. There I told another woman, 'I'm having a hard time getting through all these side effects.' She said, 'I have a friend who is getting involved with a Breast Cancer Coalition group in town. You might want to call her, because she's looking for other women to talk to.' It turned out to be Nancy Johnson. We became each other's support."

Roberta's faith in God and her husband, Dominic, were her main sources of emotional support during her illness and treatment. Although her chemotherapy treatment lasted six months, her ordeal with breast cancer ended up stretching over nearly ten years. Like the other women, she tried to keep her life as normal as possible by continuing to work full-time and maintaining her personal life. She scheduled her chemo treatments so that she could recuperate over weekends.

"I had a few strange religious moments happen during this time," she says. "I really believe in prayer. I never ask for things, just for guidance, and I usually get it. I had been wanting to go to this nearby Lutheran church and Dominic and I finally went after my surgery. They had a laying on of hands and I started bawling. But I couldn't make myself go up there and say the words, 'I have cancer.' Dominic said, 'It's not that man up there who's doing the healing. Just pray.'

"I began to pray and stopped crying instantly. There was a huge cross hanging free over the altar. As I opened my eyes in the middle of my prayer, a purple light came down from the center of the cross onto me. I didn't tell anyone about it then. I figured everybody's going to think that I've really lost it; this chemotherapy has really done some damage. Later, I told a couple of friends who are very religious and they said that people who have had healing experiences often have described a similar experience. I was pretty excited about that.

"Then I started having extremely negative visions whenever I drove to work or anywhere else: visions of me in the hospital, of Dominic and family around me crying, other horrible thoughts. I began to be afraid to drive because of these persistent visions. One Sunday morning, I decided to go to church by myself and found that they were having another laying on of hands. God was giving me a second chance. I stood up and it was as though I were walking in slow motion to the altar. I said, 'I've been diagnosed with cancer.' The ministers, a young couple, laid their hands on my head and my shoulders and prayed over me. I felt the heat from their hands. I went back to my seat, crying. During the five-minute drive from my house to the church that morning, I'd had those horrible visions. After the laying on of hands, I got in my car and never had another thought or vision like that again. I was healed of my fears."

After Roberta's six months of chemo, her husband decided to leave his position as a stockbroker to become a thoroughbred horse trainer. "We were broker than broke because we were putting all our money in the business," says Roberta. "It was hard, dealing with the chemo and being strapped for money all the time. I did all the stress reduction things you're supposed to do. I also did Domy's bookkeeping and worked at Merrill Lynch full-time."

Roberta asked her doctor for a bone scan in December 1989, two years after her initial treatment. Her doctor refused. "I told him that my other doctor had said that I should have one after a couple of years. This doctor said, 'You're asymptomatic and I don't do that.' So I didn't do it."

What she did do, in the meantime, was bring a successful lawsuit against the breast clinic that had originally misdiagnosed her mammogram. As a result, the doctor there had his license revoked and the clinic was shut down. "We didn't do it for money. We did it to get it on the books, in case other women were misdiagnosed," says Roberta. "Then we closed that chapter in our lives and went back to work on starting a family. About two months later, I began to get back pains."

This time, the doctor agreed to do a bone scan. "I'm thinking that everything will be fine; it's been two-and-a-half years and my other doctor had said that most recurrences happen in the first two years," says Roberta. "Dominic and I had started house hunting and had found one we liked. We had stopped to have a burger when I remembered that I was supposed to call the doctor to get the results of the bone scan. I called him from the restaurant and he told me, 'We found something that looks like cancer.' I dropped the phone, ran out to the car and just screamed.

"Dominic and I went home, sat on the couch, held each other and cried. Every time I'd start to feel happy, to feel as if I could get on with my life, I'd get slammed down again. Growing up, all I ever wanted in life was a home and children. The cancer was costing me my dream and, now, very possibly my life."

The doctor told Roberta that the cancer had returned in her seventh thoracic (T7) vertebra. He prescribed Tamoxifen, a drug that suppresses the effects of estrogen and inhibits cell growth. A subsequent magnetic resonance imaging (MRI) exam revealed that the cancer already had eaten away about three-quarters of her vertebra.

"I still wanted a biopsy, to be one hundred percent certain," says Roberta. "We had a hard time finding a doctor who would do it. I am so petite and everything is so compact in that area— T7 is between the shoulder blades, and my heart, lung and spinal cord are all right there. We finally found a surgeon who agreed to do it. He had to go in from the back, remove a few inches of my rib so he could get his hand in there and hold my heart away while he biopsied the tissue."

Afterward, the surgeon and his assistant sewed her up and left a guide needle inside her back. Roberta woke up on the operating table, hearing the two doctors arguing. "One said, 'Let's just let her go back to her room. The needle isn't anyplace that will be hazardous. After she recuperates, we can go back in and take it out.' The other said, 'No, I know this woman. She's going to want it taken out now.' I decided to put in my two cents and said, 'Just take it out, *now*,' and scared the hell out of both of them. They didn't know I was awake. So they put me back under and took out the needle."

Following her back surgery, Roberta had radiation every other day for four months. "It was the worst recuperation of all my surgeries," she recounts. "I had to be put on morphine for the first time in my life. I got off that right away and instead went to an acupuncturist every other day. I did a lot of holistic things to reduce the pain and stress, including visualization, meditation, cleansing my chakras. I worked on surviving day by day. And I worked full-time. During the following year, I had several more MRI tests. I also had severe blurring of vision and tingling in my legs. It was a year before I felt fully recovered.

"My sister and a good friend both offered to be surrogate mothers for us. I always wanted to have Dominic's kids; I thought he was so talented and multi-faceted. I asked the doctor, 'How does Tamoxifen affect my eggs?' He said, 'Wait a second, we don't want to get into that. That's a whole other topic. You shouldn't think about it for at least two years.' I said, 'We're not talking about doing it now, we're talking two years down the line, whatever it takes.' He replied, 'We're talking about single parenting now. There's more cancer there; we're just not seeing it yet.'

"Dominic hit the wall. He told the doctor, 'Nobody thinks about their spouse's mortality when they're thinking about children. Anybody could get hit by a bus.' The doctor said, 'Well, the chances of getting hit by a bus are pretty slim, and that's not the situation here.'

"I fired that doctor. I don't expect an oncologist to give me hope, but I do expect him to allow me the hope that I've been holding onto. I found another doctor, and he allowed me that hope. He asked me, 'Has anyone ever given you your prognosis?' I said, 'No.' He said, 'Well, if ever you're ready to hear it, let me know.' I never have asked. That was in 1990."

After that, Roberta and Dominic took every day as it came. "I knew that the doctors give you an average of two years after a recurrence," says Roberta. "I wanted to do all I could to get more focus on this disease, to help other women. I joined a support group study that Stanford University was doing on metastasized breast cancer. The members of this group all viewed breast cancer as a chronic condition. It might flare up in your hip, your back, in your lungs. It seemed everyone in the group had had multiple recurrences. I was one of the few people who'd had only one recurrence.

"Two years later, in 1992, I got a pain in my abdomen that doubled me over. It gradually went away, but then returned about three months later. I went to my regular doctor and he diagnosed a spastic colon. My mom has the same condition, so at first I accepted that. Then I got to thinking that with my history, I'd better be more careful. So I went back to my oncologist.

"I was still taking Tamoxifen, still having hot flashes and still having my periods regularly, which the doctors found unbelievable. Between chemo and Tamoxifen, your periods usually shut down. The doctor decided to do a computerized axial tomography (CAT) scan. It revealed a grapefruit-sized cyst on my ovary. The doctor said that this was a common thing to have. Actually, I was relieved! Everything else I had been through the doctors had pronounced, 'Very unusual for a girl your age.'

"I got opinions from several doctors. Two recommended a total hysterectomy. Two others recommended removing only the ovaries. I did some research on my own and found that there was some controversy about Tamoxifen and uterine wall cancer. Since my ovaries were shot anyway, I decided to have them take everything out. It was a breeze of a surgery compared to the others. They biopsied some lymph nodes and tissue they had removed and found no traces of cancer."

The hysterectomy marked the end of Roberta's dream of having children of her own. But her ordeal with breast cancer strengthened her more than she realized for the challenge of Aconcagua.

Reconstruction

THE ASCENT BACK TO HEALTH and a normal life after surgery and treatment for breast cancer is a daunting task that often requires putting one's life back in order—often, a new order, with a different set of priorities. The fact that cancer has invaded one's body remains an ever-present awareness, and leaves many women teetering on a frightful precipice. Andrea Martin explains the feeling: "The least little pain in your abdomen, the flu, a cold, an ache, and you're struck with fright again. You think you have cancer again; you're going to die. It's a struggle to maintain focus on the present, on little things that bring joy and hope."

Patty started having back pain about a year after her treatment and was certain that it must be uterine cancer. "They say that taking Tamoxifen can increase the risk of uterine cancer, but the

117

real story is that you would have gotten uterine cancer anyway," she states. "The Tamoxifen just makes it show up sooner. So because I'm on Tamoxifen, every time I get this pain, I worry that it's a recurrence. I've had tests done, x-rays taken, and I'm fine. It's with me every day. I try and put it out of my mind."

Kim has been on and off Tamoxifen. "I took it for a year after my treatment, then stopped because we thought we'd try to have kids again," she says. "I told myself, if I wasn't pregnant by the time I reached forty, I'd go back on again. I didn't get pregnant, so I started Tamoxifen again. I'm not crazy about the side effects, such as breakthrough bleeding, feeling a little depression, feeling a little muddled at times."

The drug has had a different effect on Sara, who had no radiation or chemotherapy after her mastectomy. She takes two Tamoxifen every morning, and feels great. "I feel better than I've ever felt in my life. I can't figure it out, but I like it. When I give talks, my message is, 'Life may not begin at sixty, but it doesn't end at sixty, either.'"

The effects of treatment and medication prematurely thrust many of the women into menopause, complete with cessation of menstrual periods and the onset of hot flashes, vaginal dryness and decreased libido. Some of the younger women eventually regained their menstrual cycles and shed the effects of menopause. The others remained in menopause.

"The bottom line in this early menopause stuff is that it comes on so quickly, unlike normal menopause," says Andrea Martin. "You lose your libido suddenly. It's like having amnesia. You wake up one morning and something important in your life is suddenly gone. Once I got on Tamoxifen, I dried up. So how do you get your life back? I haven't found any chemical or cream on the market that restores the libido. You simply have to make an extra effort and hope that your spouse or boyfriend is understanding."

It takes a strong and flexible relationship to withstand the attack of a vicious adversary like cancer. For several of the women, cancer precipitated the end of a marriage or intimate relationship. For others, cancer became a catalyst for strengthening or renewing a relationship. Reentering society as a single-breasted, no-breasted or partially-breasted woman also presented a challenge, one that involved adjusting to a different perspective of self-image, body-awareness and sexuality. Indeed, as each woman discovered, the words, *breast cancer survivor*, encompassed more than thwarting a life-threatening disease.

Andrea Martin says she didn't "hold back many punches" with her daughter, Mather. "Who knows if that was the right approach? At least she knows what is going on; she knows that friends have died of this disease. She knows that I have taken death in stride. I made a conscious effort not to scare the bejeezus out of her, but I want her to be able to face reality. I tried to maintain some sense of normalcy. I survived. That's the bottom line."

Roberta survived her treatments, but her marriage didn't. In 1993, less than two years after her hysterectomy, Roberta and Dominic reached an impasse. "Dominic couldn't handle the stress," reflects Roberta. "He had been great up until then. I now believe that he was brought into my life to help take care of me, to help me heal. A couple of years after we separated, he told me that when I had the recurrence in my back, he had made a pact with God: that if I didn't have to ever deal with cancer again, he would give up whatever he considered to be the most precious thing to him. He said that about a year after my hysterectomy, he realized that the thing that was most precious was me.

"He knew he was extremely unreliable and irresponsible. I never really realized the stress he was putting me through until he was gone. My friends used to say, 'How can you live with this man? He's so exasperating and frustrating.' Our life together was a real roller-coaster ride. He'd make a success of something, then tear it down, self-destruct, and go on to something else. We were either riding high or on the verge of bankruptcy. I used to tell him that I'd stick by him no matter what, except if he had an affair. And that's what he did."

After Roberta confronted Dominic and his girlfriend, Dominic moved out. "The girl left her husband, but she and Domy eventually broke it off," says Roberta. "It was rough. When I was going through all that other pain, it was some outside force causing the pain and I had him to hold onto. Now, not only did I not have him to hold onto but it was Domy, whom I loved most, who was causing me the pain. It took me a couple of years to adjust."

Roberta plunged into fundraising work for the Breast Cancer Fund and eventually became a member of its board. "After selling tickets for one fundraiser, Andrea Martin asked me to be on the steering committee for a fashion show fundraiser," says Roberta. "I thought it might be a good diversion for me, so I agreed. She also asked me to model. Then I found out that I was to be the finale, *the bride*. It was so ironic. But it turned out to be a good experience and really pulled me out of a place that I could have easily gone, wallowing in misery."

Roberta began to realize that she was now able to live her life for herself. "With Dominic, all of my dreams were on the back burner. He'd say, 'Hang in there, sweetie, you'll get your dreams, I promise you.' Since we ended the marriage, I've learned to make myself first. I've always been the type of person to say, 'Oh no, I can't do that.' I was such a contradiction because I loved the gamble, the excitement of being with Domy and watching him take risks, but I was never going to take any risks myself. When I was growing up, my idea of a failure was if you tried something and it failed—then you're a failure. If you don't try anything, I thought, then you're not a failure. So I never tried anything."

Vicki and Larry's relationship also crumbled under the weight of cancer. A few nights before her mastectomy, they made love for what turned out to be the last time. "I cried the whole time," says Vicki. "Larry had helped me through decisions, he was there for me, but it wore him out. During chemo, I felt kind of androgynous. All I wanted to wear was big T-shirts and baggy pants. I felt as if I had lost my femininity. It wasn't until chemo was over and I started to come back into myself that I began to realize that I still had the feminine profile on one side, but my other side looked like a boy. Then I started to play with the whole femininity-in-your-breast issue. By the time I started wanting some loving again, I figured he'd been waiting for me all that time. Instead, he had shut down.

"One night, I asked Larry, 'Does my body turn you off?' He wouldn't answer me. I stood there with my shirt off and asked him, 'Do you have a hard time seeing this? Do you think it's ugly?' He finally said, 'I don't know if I would actually call it ugly.' Then he cried and said that he felt awful.

"He finally told me that he wanted to break up with me, that he had actually been thinking of it before I was diagnosed with cancer. The day I was diagnosed, he said, he decided that he would stick with me through the chemo, then leave.

"That angered me. I said, 'You've been marking off the calendar all this time, waiting for me to be emotionally strong enough for you to leave?' At that point, I wished he had left in the beginning."

Like many of the other women, during her illness Vicki had been forced to focus solely on herself, on her needs, to survive.

In the meantime, Larry was struggling with his own feelings and fears. "I realized later that Larry has had a lot of cancer in his life," says Vicki. "A college friend had died of lymphoma, a girl-friend died of ovarian cancer, his father died of leukemia. So when Larry looks at my scar, he sees cancer. I see life and he sees cancer. He would never talk to me about it."

Annette also got an I-had-been-thinking-of-breaking-up-with-you message from her boyfriend. They had been dating for about a year when she was diagnosed. Theirs was a long-distance relationship, in more ways than one. "He lived in Los Angeles. I lived in Seattle. But he came up four or five times during the eight months of my treatment," recalls Annette. "He was here for two of the chemo treatments. When I started to lose my hair, he helped me shave my head. Afterwards, we had an incredibly tender, loving and passionate lovemaking session.

"After my treatments were finished, I went to Los Angeles and I was thinking how, after having gone through this negative experience, things were going to be wonderful between us. Instead, he told me, 'You know, I don't want you to take this the wrong way, but before you were diagnosed I really was thinking about leaving the relationship. I never wanted to act on it because I knew that you wouldn't let me be part of this experience with you.'

"I was so angry. I told him, 'I didn't need a nurse. I needed a friend.' We broke up for a while and then got back together. We were off and on for about two years. At first, I couldn't accept the fact that we'd gone through all this together and weren't going to build on it. He was there for some important moments and not for others. Unable to make a commitment."

For Annette, this became another lesson gleaned from the cancer experience. "You do your best and then you let go," she says. "Make a decision and then move on. Let go of knowing the outcome beforehand."

Sue Anne felt she could not let go of her marriage because, she says, "I wasn't self-sufficient." Cancer added another dimension of separateness between Sue Anne and her husband. "When I got my diagnosis and went through a period of hitting bottom, Gary hugged me but he seemed immobilized and depressed himself. My backyard is full of trees and has always been a comfort. I'd often go outside and park myself in nature."

Sue Anne's struggle with depression was, in some ways, more difficult than her cancer ordeal, she believes. "When you have cancer, you get a lot of support. Most people can identify with it. Depression is more elusive. With depression, people think you can snap out of it. It's not that way at all."

A "gift" finally came in answer to Sue Anne's earlier circle-of-chairs cry for help. At a Noetic Science meeting, she met a man who put her in touch with his sister, a healer who lived in St. Louis. "At first, I thought, 'St. Louis?' but then I got that same intuitive feeling at the base of my neck when I first thought that I might have cancer. So I agreed to call her.

"She called me back with an assignment. For twenty minutes before I went to sleep at night and before I got up in the morning, I was to put my hands over my breasts and then, for twenty more minutes, over my ovaries. I asked, 'Do I breathe or visualize?' She said, 'Do nothing but put your hands there, be still, and I will do the same from here.'

"I did this for three or four weeks. Then she called and said that she was coming to California to see her new grandchild and would come and stay with me as long as I needed her. I had taken in people and pets, I had shared our home with a Russian family for over nine months, which had added stress to our family. At first I could hear all the voices of people around me: 'Who is she? Why would she do this? How much is it going to cost?'

"She showed up and gave me treatments and cooked with me. It was so wonderful to have someone to eat with, because most of the time I would eat outside on the patio by myself. And I would experience grief, because all the time I would be thinking, 'Why is this happening to me?' This woman was here for eight days, and did Reiki treatments on me several times a day. *Reiki* is the Japanese word for universal life force energy. It's a way to balance inner and outer realities. Two or three times a day, I'd lie on the massage table. She put her hands on me, but she didn't massage. She would leave her hands there longer if she felt more energy coming. She was very intuitive. It was the first time I had felt such stillness.

"I had chemo while she was here. Usually, I spin and spin in multiple circles and layers and keep myself so distracted that I don't get to the core of things. I'm really good at that. Her treatments were a quieting experience that stopped me in my tracks. I finally got still enough to look at my life, my choices, my options, my feelings. I started to learn to say *no*. I used to never say no to anyone. I felt if something came to me to do, then I should do it.

"We'd sit up late and talk, purge the confusion. She did Reiki on the kids, too, and they loved it. It was a nice change from all the disruption and disintegration in the house. She was the first one on the scene from a totally alien source, not from my circle of friends. A friend of mine commented, 'This is like you, to have your angels in the flesh.'

"Then she was gone. But it was as though I had received a jump start. I continued to go to the Noetic Science meetings. This group seemed to be a filter factor to find kindred souls. The healer's message stayed with me: be still.

"At one of the meetings, I met an anthropologist who was also a drummer. We'd sit in circles while he drummed. It was fascinating, captivating and revealing. At one session, I sat there with my eyes closed and heard chanting with the drumming. I wondered how he could drum and chant at the same time. At the end, I asked who was chanting and people looked at me so funny. I was the only one who had heard it. I thought, 'Okay, that will be my little gift tonight.' I was learning to receive inner gifts in whatever way they came to me. It was very humbling."

As Sue Anne gained strength, she continued to try to understand her relationship with Gary. "I had always been active, but my husband listened to a different drummer. He likes to stay at home and keep to himself. Originally, I was attracted to him because of his quiet, kind manner. He's sensitive to nature, good with animals and a good artist. But the very qualities that drew me to him began to separate us. Our inability to work through and process life together was a great sadness. In sickness and in health—something was missing here. At first, I couldn't comprehend it. Then, when I finally did comprehend it, I couldn't accept it. Then, when I finally accepted it, I didn't know what to do. I wanted to escape, but something made me stay. I got to a place where I was able to give up expectations and flow with whatever life delivered. I stopped feeling that I had to fix everyone else. Someone said we are healed not by what we turn from but what we turn toward. I started learning to mind my own business while gaining the realization that we are all one."

Kim underwent many changes during her cancer experience, at the expense of her relationship. "Cancer became a powerful test of the strength of our marriage," she reflects. Art had lost his parents at a young age and now was faced with the possibility of losing his wife. He was consumed by his feelings, and at times became bitter towards Kim. "We not only had a new baby, we also had cancer. We had no time to sit back and digest all that had happened. Suddenly, things just weren't the way they used to be, or the way we expected them to be. Suddenly, our reality was so different than the day before we found out we had cancer.

"To Art, to be able to admit that the cancer was hard on him was a sign of weakness. He was angry at the powers that be; he was angry at me. This wasn't in his game plan. Cancer caused us to get into some bad habits, like not talking to each other, not dealing with our emotions. I found that my friends were better to talk to. Art was so stoic and tightlipped about the whole thing. I'd have had a lot more respect for him if he'd told me that he was having trouble with it. At one point, I wondered if this was just the way men deal with things, as opposed to the way women deal with things. I don't know.

"I think the stronger I get, the harder it is for him. He sees me getting stronger from the cancer, excelling in some things careerwise, getting involved in other things. He says, 'You've changed since we got married.' I say, 'Thank God, look at all the changes that have happened in our lives. I'm not going to be static.' All this change began as a result of cancer. I see change as growth, not as a bad thing. Change intimidates Art; he can't deal with it, can't talk about it. We live in a state of ambivalence."

One of the team members started taking estrogen because, she said, "I was beginning to feel like a neuter. You know, you desperately need someone to put their arms around you and love you and tell you that you're okay—any time of your life, whether you're twenty-five or eighty-five. With menopause, you have all these hormonal changes, vaginal dryness, your desire for sex diminishes on top of being more tired. Unless you have had a wonderful relationship beforehand, it's difficult to talk about. Instead, my husband would say, 'You're not interested' or 'You're not sexy' because he didn't want to be the one who was rejected.

And I started to believe it.

"I tried to get my husband to see a counselor with me. I got all the literature and there was a medication they were testing that I even considered trying, but my husband wouldn't have anything to do with it. Intimacy is our problem, but I am the one causing the problem, according to his perspective.

"After I came off chemotherapy, I was dealing with a lot of fear. One morning at breakfast, I told my husband about it, about how worried and upset I was, and how low I felt. He listened to me, then turned and looked outside and said, 'Do you think we need to cut the grass today?' I had to leave the table. He realized what he'd done but he couldn't do anything about it. In the beginning of a marriage, you're so ready to share. I was ready to share my soul, but then I finally realized that I wasn't getting any of that back. When that sort of thing keeps happening over a long period of time, you stop. Then you establish a different kind of relationship."

For Sara and Fritz, cancer strengthened an already comfortable marriage. "We've been happily married since 1956," says Sara, "and we've grown at the same pace. I married Fritz after I graduated from Smith. Adlai Stevenson spoke at the graduation ceremony and told us, 'Go out and be good wives and mothers.' Today, this guy would be drummed right out of politics and off the face of the earth. Back then, that's what I heard and that's what I swallowed—and that's what I've been.

"Meeting Fritz was the greatest, luckiest thing that ever happened to me. But I think when you have a scare, whether it's cancer or any other close call, all of a sudden you wake up and say, 'Holy cow, I'm *really* lucky.' The cancer strengthened our relationship. He's been so much more attentive and loving, I'm almost afraid to talk about it for fear it will all just go away."

Laura and her husband, Roger, had enjoyed a very active sex

life before her illness and treatment. In her testimonial book, *The Climb of My Life*, she describes the frustration they both endured. "I was so thankful to be out of the hospital...for Roger's strong arms, which wrapped around me with loving hugs. But...I wanted to take myself back in time, before all this happened. I cried for what was lost—for the familiar life, for the old me, the long-haired, blond, wild and crazy me....

"I didn't understand, then, that I was in the middle of a process, the process required to get through any crisis.... The body and mind required time to heal, to sort things out.... I would have to work through this slowly, much as I used to climb mountains, one step at a time." Eventually, with patience and understanding, the intimacy they had enjoyed was restored. Laura wrote, "We would rebuild our lives together, finding new common ground, a new way to be lovers."

Andrea Martin's marriage was also strengthened, although she acknowledges that it could have gone the other way. "Cancer takes a toll. The sexuality part is really key. It's all wrapped up in the physiology of the treatment, the psychology of losing a breast and going through other kinds of surgery, the shattering of your security. People talk about 'damaged goods.' Sharing all this with a partner or trying to incorporate it if you date or see other people or eventually hope to is difficult.

"When I was diagnosed, I was very into sex and in a new relationship with a wonderful partner. And all of a sudden my desire was gone. During that year of chemo, my body went through so many changes, but Richard very lovingly and kindly refused to let me roll up and die. He kept us sexually active without imposing himself on me. But after chemo ended, it took me over a year to begin to feel the energy and vitality I had before I got sick.

"First, I used testosterone cream. Then I started taking testosterone in daily capsules, and it gave me a slight hint of what I used to feel. Then it plateaued. So we found ways to get me turned on in a new way. It's like learning how to walk again. For a long time, once I got into sex, it was great, but I couldn't initiate it. In fact, I felt if I never had sex again, it would be okay. All of that has changed, and it's been an incredible journey. Richard and I have learned *tantra,* the art of conscious lovemaking. But getting here took real desire and hard work. It also took a man who was in love with me, not with my breasts."

Patty and her husband, Peter, also had to make some adjustments. "I'm totally dry and there's nothing on the market that really works, that makes you moist," says Patty. "There are suppositories that work for three days. Oh yeah, I'm going to use this and be wet for three days. I don't think so. If you really love someone, there are ways to make it all work."

Claudia Berryman-Shafer, whose marriage was strong before, during and after her surgery and chemo, but who has witnessed the effects of cancer on her friends' relationships, offers this succinct observation: "It seems that husbands or boyfriends of women with breast cancer are either very supportive, or jerks."

Another issue that the women with mastectomies had to deal with was whether or not to undergo reconstruction. Nancy Johnson, Andrea Martin, Mary, Patty, Claudia Berryman-Shafer, Vicki, Sara and Sue Anne elected not to have reconstruction done.

Sara never considered it. "My marriage is not going to dissolve over a breast," she says. "Physicians won't do it anyway if you're over seventy, and I'm close enough, so who the heck cares!"

Claudia Crosetti had the tramflap reconstruction done at the same time as her mastectomy, but the procedure did not include nipple reconstruction. "That's done later and I just never got around to it," she says. "I don't want another surgery."

Patty agrees. "The way I look at it," she says, "I've had two cesareans and I opted during the second one to tie my tubes because I didn't want to go through that operation again. I tried the SOB—that's what I call the Stick-On-Boob prosthesis—and it was more trouble than it was worth. I'd stick it in there and start walking and it would end up down by my stomach. Or I'd get a rash from it. You have to wear a special kind of bra so that it won't fall out when you bend over, and I don't even like to wear bras. I finally decided, 'Screw it.' I don't mind going out in a bathing suit with one boob sticking out. It doesn't bother me and it doesn't bother Peter. He says, 'Here's winking at you,' because that's what the scar reminds him of, a wink."

Eleanor wore a prosthesis for a year, during her chemotherapy. "My husband used to refer to me as Little Wingy, because I only had one wing. He told me that he loved me and was very concerned for me, but I think it made him uncomfortable."

After her second mastectomy, Eleanor had reconstruction of both breasts. "I didn't want to wear two prostheses," she says. "It's too uncomfortable and I didn't want to go without having any breasts at all. For some women, that's okay. I think it has to do with how comfortable you are with your body."

Nancy Hudson planned to have reconstruction at some point in the near future. "After five years with one breast, I want something that looks natural, so I can put clothes on," she explained. "I don't like having to think about it all the time. I don't like being in dressing rooms with anybody else. I don't feel whole. I mean, I have this big, twelve-inch scar on one side and a pancake on the other. The doctors said I'd have to have them both done so that they'd look even. It's an easy operation, but it's tough to think about going back under again. But I think it would help me feel better about myself."

Like Claudia Crosetti and Ashley, Roberta had breast reconstruction right after her mastectomy. "I fought with the doctors to have a skin expander put in at the time the mastectomy was done because I wanted to eliminate more surgical procedure," she says. A skin expander is a temporary implant placed under the skin and injected with saline, once a week in Roberta's case, to stretch out the skin. "I didn't have enough tissue anywhere else on my body to use for reconstruction. They overstretch the skin so that when they finally put in the permanent implant, it will be more supple and look more natural."

Roberta was angry at Dominic for plunging her into the singles' world. "I hadn't dated since high school and now, suddenly, dating took on a whole new significance. How and when do you approach the subject of breast cancer? There are lots of books and articles about breast cancer, surgery, treatment, support groups and even advice for the married woman—but nothing for the single woman." The answer came to Roberta in a very unexpected and joyful way, through her relationship with Kipp. When she finally showed him her breast, he got down on his knees before her and tenderly kissed the scar. "It was hard not to fall for him after that," she said.

Annette also didn't think about the implications of breast cancer on her sexuality until she started dating a new man. "I never thought about mentioning it at first," she says. "We had gone kayaking and were having a beer. He asked me if I wanted to do something next. I said, 'Well, I have to go run stairs.' And as soon as I said it, I realized that it sounded like, you know, 'I have to go paint my toenails or put my hair up in curlers—anything rather than go out on a date with you.' I told him, 'Actually, I need to explain about these stairs.' I told him that I was training for a climb. It was a climb for breast cancer and involved breast cancer survivors—like me! I was hesitant, because cancer still makes some people a little freaky. This guy didn't know anything, whether I'd had a lumpectomy or mastectomy or what my status was or anything else. He just said, 'That explains it.' 'Explains what?' I said. He said there was a real sense of inner peace and strength about me and he had wondered what it was."

Annette laughs and adds, "I think part of it was a line. But it worked. It happened at the right time and was a wonderful reaffirmation of my femininity. It was a great relationship for a few months, then became inconsistent. I really live in the moment, and that's hard for some people to understand."

Claudia Crosetti explains how her focus changed during and after treatment. "Sex was suddenly not important to me. What was important was getting through surgery and chemo and the coming year. Taking care of myself became my priority. I was getting eleven hours of sleep a night just to keep myself well rested. After chemo, I started taking Tamoxifen and went into total depression and hot flashes before it started leveling out. I was bald. And it's not only the hair on your head that you lose, you know. My eyebrows, eyelashes, pubic hairs—all gone. I looked strange and felt strange. My boyfriend, Jim, was really supportive and pretty cool, but I wanted to pamper myself and take care of myself and not think about anybody else. After my treatment ended and I started feeling better, I wanted to explore my 'new' life in a different way. Jim and I ended up breaking up several months later, but remained friends."

Claudia's period had stopped while she was on chemotherapy, then restarted after her treatments ended. "It was a monumental day," she says. "May 15, 1992. I was sitting at my desk at work and I was wearing my wig, which I hated. It itched. I got really loose with it. People would walk by and I'd rub my whole scalp and leave the wig lopsided. I hated it. I didn't even like turbans because they felt so confining.

"Anyway, it was a spring day, about a month and a half after my chemo had ended. I had started my period that day, and somebody at work said, 'Why don't you take off the wig and leave it off?' So I did. I had a little buzz of hair covering my head. Spring had sprung and here I am with some hair and my period. It was like a rebirth for me, as if I were part of the cycle of the earth."

The cancer experience ultimately bonded the relationship between Nancy Johnson and her partner, Janet. But, as Nancy explains, "We definitely went through some challenging times around it spiritually, physically and emotionally. It was a challenge to cope with the differences. Physically, I had a whole different body. I felt really strange. I wondered, 'Am I still going to be sexually pleasing to this person without my breasts?' Janet was an incredible support through the whole episode. I can't imagine going through it without her."

Nevertheless, the combination of having cancer, turning forty and losing her father the following year produced in Nancy a need for independence. "Through my illness, I redefined my priorities," she says. "I also went through a stage where I felt as if I had to start doing everything because I thought my life was going to end soon. I had faced my own mortality and then, three months after my surgery, my father died of cancer. That plunged me into a morbid, depressed place. First I had lost my breasts and then my father. He and I had been very close. I had a difficult time accepting the loss. It reminded me of how short life is, and how we tend to take good health for granted."

After her treatment, Ashley left Charlottesville seeking a healthier and more independent environment. "I was tired of people talking to my chest," she states. "I was tired of being the youngest girl in Charlottesville ever to get breast cancer." She moved to Missoula and enrolled in the University of Montana as a psychology major. The move lessened her notoriety, until she became a team member.

"There were articles about me in our local newspaper, so eventually everyone at school and in town knew," she says. "As it turned out, it was a great way to get dates. Guys would come up to me and ask, 'Have you gone on the climb yet?' And I didn't have to go through the whole breast cancer story because they already knew. They'd read about me. It sort of separated the good ones from the bad. The ones who wanted to be with me said that knowing what had happened to me made me more desirable because, you know—*strength.*"

It still didn't make sex easier, Ashley acknowledges. "I've got scars everywhere—from my reduction, from the mastectomy, from the reconstruction. When I first was with boys in college, we'd have sex and I'd burst into tears and I'd go get in the shower by myself and cry and not understand why. I told one guy that breast cancer was not a part of me and we ignored it. When we had sex, he ignored my breasts. That didn't feel right, either. It's a hard thing to deal with."

Nancy Hudson agrees. "Losing a breast is a big deal. You've got two legs, two arms and you are supposed to have two breasts. The first time you expose yourself to someone, it's a huge step. I dated two different guys who were so supportive. It didn't bother them at all. They'd say, 'It's what's going on in your head and heart that I like.' One of the guys would even rub my scar, which made me feel self-conscious. It's me. I'm the one who's bothered by it all."

After her cancer treatment and reconstruction, Eleanor decided to go through hospice training to explore her own death and life. "I wanted to know, 'Where do I stand on this? Can I be more comfortable with it?'" she says. "I had come face-to-face with my mortality, but was I comfortable with dying? Or with people around me dying? During training, one of the exercises we did was to take a blank sheet of paper and draw our spirituality.

"I thought about it for a while and then I drew a great big tree with leaves reaching to the ground and a very full crown. In the tree were my children and my husband, and the roots to the ground, I realized, were my motherhood. I sensed of myself that this family gathered its nourishment from the ground, from the heart. And maybe I was the heart and gave the nourishment to the people in the branches. I'm a nurturing person. That's my spirituality.

"When I was on chemotherapy, I read an article in the paper about a young man who had leukemia or some kind of cancer. He was walking across the United States to raise money and awareness. His feet were all bloody; he was having a difficult time. People were following him. I marveled at his story. During that time, somebody called me and asked me to be the chairperson for a fundraising event at University of the Arts in Philadelphia. I'd never done anything like that. I'd always been a mother, working or in school. I thought to myself, 'Why are they calling me?' I read this article and I thought, 'You know what, Eleanor? This is a wake-up call. What do you have to lose? Try it. You might enjoy it.' And I did. And now I'm on the board of that college, and I've met so many wonderful people."

Eleanor has a hard time being called a "survivor." She dislikes the terminology. "People die of this disease, and what do you call them, the non-survivors?" she says. "What do I get, a special medal for surviving? I don't know exactly how to get it across, but we're lucky. We're the fortunate ones. We're veterans. If we could find a cure, we'd all be here, we'd all be veterans.

"I deal with so many women in the work I do with hospice

and bereavement counseling, and with the American Cancer Society. I see this incredible spirit in women, this incredible spirit about their families, about their husbands, about their children. They want to be there for them. They want to make life easier for them. They will get through this—they will somehow *survive* as long as they can and make the best of it. It's not about survival as much as it is about the resiliency of the human spirit. I see it time and again with the cancer diagnosis. And I marvel at it. I marvel at the resiliency of the human spirit."

Like Eleanor, the other women emerged from their cancer ordeals wanting to somehow give back, to lend support to other women afflicted with the disease and to raise awareness in all women about the importance of taking charge of their health and their lives. Expedition Inspiration gave them that opportunity.

Shortly before leaving for Argentina, Nancy Johnson explained, "The way I look at it, I gave up my breasts to be here. I love life. I'm pretty greedy for life. Looking back on the experience, it wasn't that difficult a thing to do so that I could be here. I chose to live with my scars, to not have any reconstruction or wear a prosthesis. I've adjusted well to that. In fact, my scars remind me every day that this is why I'm alive.

"I also decided early on in my experience with breast cancer that I didn't want to become yet another silence. I didn't want to contribute to the silent epidemic. So I started learning more and talking more. I couldn't believe how little I knew about this disease when I first got it and how much I had learned by the following year. I felt I had an obligation. I wanted to tell everybody: 'Did you know you can get it at any age?' 'Don't let this happen to you.' 'Do you realize you don't have to find a lump to have cancer?' 'Are you getting mammograms?' 'Are you relying only on self-exam?' I felt I had to tell people this stuff.

What if people were dying right now because I hadn't told them? I felt it was my duty and responsibility to protect my friends. I'm sure part of it was anger, too. I was angry because so little has been done to arrest this disease. I wanted somehow to play a role. So I helped start the Breast and Cervical Cancer Control Program in our community. That's when I met Claudia Crosetti, and we went on to organize a walk-a-thon to raise awareness and funds, but also to bring together other women in the community who had the disease."

Nancy added, "It made us realize how much this disease has touched people's lives and how hungry people are to have an opportunity to talk about it or just have the subject brought up. I knew right then I was going to spend a lot of time in my life doing stuff like this. It's so important, so needed and so rewarding. To be a part of Expedition Inspiration was an incredible opportunity to raise awareness on a national level."

For Claudia B–S, the expedition also came along at the right time. "Jim and I are both teachers and we work with a large female population. Women have come up to both of us and said, 'I've never had a mammogram. If somebody like Claudia can get this, then I can, too.' So that awareness has been increased. And the awareness among kids, too, spread at our school. I mean, before you didn't even say the word, *breast*, in sixth grade. But my sixth grade class and really, the whole school, wanted to know everything about the surgery and the chemotherapy, so I told them. I explained everything—what is breast cancer, what do they do about it, what is chemo like. It's been real neat to talk to kids about it. I've had kids come up and whisper to me, 'My mom had the same kind of cancer that you have.' I say, 'Breast cancer?' 'Yeah,' they nod. This kind of awareness is the most important thing that has come about as the result of my cancer."

Claudia adds, "The other important thing that happened was

to be with the team on Rainier in July—to listen to other women and know that they were thinking the same way, had gone through the same funny stuff and the same hard stuff. I'm looking forward to the expedition in January—and it's taking so long to get here!"

Part Three

The Outward Journey

"To me, this climb is a celebration of wellness."
—Claudia Berryman-Shafer

The Ascent

O N FRIDAY, JANUARY 20, 1995, the eighteen-person
summit team of Expedition Inspiration—and its fifty-seven
duffels of gear—boarded Aerolinas Argentinas in Los Angeles,
California, for the thirteen-hour flight to Buenos Aires, Argentina. Five days later, the trek team would follow our trail.

We read, played cards, ate or slept throughout most of the
flight. Our sojourn in sprawling, cosmopolitan Buenos Aires
consisted of a bus ride from the international airport to the national airport, where we caught another, shorter flight to the
more provincial town of Mendoza.

Mendoza was home for two nights and a day while we organized gear. Peter and the guides confirmed our travel arrangements for the next leg of the trip. During our short stay, we
found Mendoza to be a delightful, tree-shaded town of friendly

people and excellent restaurant fare. Nevertheless, when the chartered bus picked us up Sunday morning for the four-hour drive to the tiny mountain hamlet of Puenta del Inca, staging point for all climbs of Aconcagua, everyone was eager to hit the road.

"I'm glad to be finally doing this instead of talking about it," said Claudia B-S, expressing the sentiment of the entire team.

In Puenta del Inca, we spent two nights at a hostel for climbers and skiers, six to a room. Meals were simple but hearty. Our minds were not on food, anyway. Although we could not see Aconcagua from the valley that cradles Puenta del Inca, the mountain's proximity reverberated throughout the hostel and the hamlet. Photographs of various climbing expeditions decorated the walls of the hostel's restaurant. The place was alive with the comings and goings of various climbing parties. Stories circulated quickly, especially those with disheartening or tragic news.

We heard more than once how inclement weather had thwarted many climbers during the previous month. One party of climbers told us that a recent storm had dumped snow at base camp and prevented several parties from advancing up the mountain. Other climbers told of a death on the mountain, injuries and more failed summit attempts.

Peter admonished us not to worry about the weather, which could be very changeable this time of year, and not to dwell on the misfortunes of other climbers. Instead, he stated, concentrate on the day at hand. "We are prepared for anything," he assured us.

To help us acclimatize and get rid of some preclimb jitters, Peter led us on a day hike several miles up and out of the valley to a ridge that opened up to a stunning vista of Aconcagua. This was our first real look at the mountain, and we were spellbound. We all agreed that Aconcagua was much more beautiful than the vision we had seen in Peter's slides. We gulped crisp mountain air as the reality check engulfed us in chills and nervous laughter.

In the distance, Aconcagua—the Stone Sentinel—stood alone, an immense fortress of rock glazed with snow and ice. Like most of the world's highest peaks, it looked neither friendly nor inviting. The popular Ruta Normal, or Normal Route, was called a "walk-up" by many mountaineers because of its gradually ascending grade. Expedition Inspiration would not be following that route. Instead, we would make our attempt via a more difficult route, one that Peter called a variation on the "Polish Glacier Route." Neither route was visible from the vantage point on the outskirts of Puenta del Inca.

Because Puenta del Inca sits at an elevation of nearly nine thousand feet, we had plenty of opportunity to begin acclimatizing. It didn't take long to explore Puenta del Inca itself. In addition to the hostel, there was a tiny grocery store, a post office and a cluster of small booths with souvenirs for sale. A short hike from the hostel led to the ruins of a spa, reachable across a bridge, or *puenta*. We later learned that Paul Simon's famous song, "Bridge Over Troubled Waters," had been inspired by his travels in this area.

A small stone church stood immediately outside the hamlet. About ten years earlier, all the surrounding homes had been destroyed by an avalanche. The church was untouched, and is therefore considered a sacred place. All the team members eventually visited the church for last minute thoughts and prayers. The evening before the team was to depart for the trail head, Annette was leaving the church and happened to look into the sky in time to see a condor circling above. She took it as a fortuitous sign.

At ten-thirty in the morning on Tuesday, January 24, Fernando Grajales, a renowned Argentine mountaineer and local outfitter, drove the summit team to the trail head for Las Vacas Valley approach to Aconcagua. We disembarked in high spirits, eager to get moving, to take the first step in a journey for which most of us had spent the last year or longer preparing. As we were pulling on our packs, someone mentioned that Las Vacas Valley translates to, "The Valley of the Cows." "It sounds like something from 'The Far Side,'" she joked. We all laughed, conjuring up visions of Gary Larsen's anthropomorphized bovines. Oddly enough, we never saw a single cow.

We were still in high spirits when, about five-and-a-half hours and eight miles later, we arrived at our first camp, Las Lenas. It had been a good first day. Claudia B-S remarked, "We're one day closer to the summit."

The hot, dry heat, seventy-five to eighty degrees this first day, took some getting used to. Most of us had come from winter climates into Argentina's summer season. The sun radiated welcome warmth after the cool morning hours, but we were all thankful for the breeze that came up around noon. In two more days, we would reach base camp, 13,800 feet and above the heat.

The trail through Las Vacas Valley meandered up and down through the gorge of the Río de Las Vacas, over loose rock and dusty scree. The trail was hard on the ankles and feet, especially with the quick pace that Peter had set. We traveled as a tight group, more like a battalion of eighteen soldiers than a hiking party. There were no laggards. We were on a mission. As Peter stated, "After four days of travel, this is a beneficial workout for you. It'll get you back in shape for climbing."

Several of the team members listened to music on Walkman stereos to relieve the monotony of the hike and to help keep their pace consistent. Music selections varied, from Annette's Bruce Springsteen to Claudia B-S's Led Zeppelin and Nine Inch Nails. Others in the group chose to listen to the rushing Río de Las

Vacas, chirping birds and the crunch of boot heels on scree.

We stopped every hour or so for a quick "maintenance break," to drink water, eat a snack and reapply sunscreen. A few times, we had to stop to wait for the film crew to either catch up or move ahead to get in position for the next shot. During these minibreaks, we'd take in the scenery: the impressive, steep walls of colorful rock rising above the river, the blue sky dotted with puffy, white clouds, the scrubby vegetation that lent patches of green to a landscape painted mostly in gradients of earth-tone reds, grays and beiges. The area is similar to the high desert in Utah: no trees, lots of scrub brush and tough grasses, vast expanses of land and sky, gaping river gorges. The Río de Las Vacas is full and rushing, and extremely cold, coming from glacial melt.

In an effort to limit and control the environmental impact of climbers trekking to base camp at Aconcagua, the Argentine government has designated three camps along Las Vacas route. The first is Las Lenas; the second, Casa de Piedras; the third, at base camp, Plaza Argentinas. At Las Lenas, tent sites consist of bare spots surrounded by low walls of loosely piled rocks, which help block the notorious winds that regularly scour this canyon. When we arrived, there was only a light breeze and we all elected to sleep out in the open in our sleeping bags. We wanted to fall asleep looking at the canopy of stars.

We reached camp about two hours ahead of the mules. With no gear to unpack, we had time on our hands. Mary, Claudia B-S and I seized the opportunity to jump in the river for a cold and quick skinny-dipping. We knew that we would have fewer opportunities to bathe fully once we began to advance up the mountain, so we grinned and "bared" it. Washing off the trail dust felt so pleasurable. When our other teammates saw us sauntering back into camp looking squeaky clean, they, too, rushed to the river.

We warmed ourselves by stretching out in the sun on a few large boulders near camp. A dark canyon wall loomed above us. A condor soared high above on the air currents. It was the first condor sighting since Puenta del Inca.

Mary said that she felt relaxed and ready for the next day, but she also was trying not to look too far ahead. "I just want to take it one day at a time, and I've made a motto for myself: 'Hydrate, eat, relax and enjoy.' I'm trying to stick to that to keep myself focused on the moment. But now and then I find myself looking toward future days."

Our reverie was interrupted by the arrival of the twenty mules and half-dozen gauchos that Peter had hired through Grajales to transport our food and gear to base camp. Each mule carried two or three duffels. Our personal duffels were marked individually. Duffels containing group gear and food were numbered for easy access by the guides. To keep a mule steady during the unloading of duffels, the gaucho tied his jacket over the mule's head to cover its eyes. When the mule was relieved of its load and pack saddle, the gaucho hobbled its front legs and then released the mule to munch the sparse grass around camp. We stood at a respectable distance to watch the whole operation before retrieving our duffels and setting up camp.

After establishing the kitchen behind a tall boulder, the guides then built low rock walls on two sides for additional shelter from the wind. Here they set up four small tables, each about the size of a card table, two for cooking and two for serving food and hot drinks to the team. The guides had their routine down pat and we were careful to stay out of their way unless asked to help. We all remarked at what a luxury it was not to have to prepare our own meals. Many of us had wilderness experience and were capable of cooking outdoors, but the guides were adamant: "Go take care of your gear, treat your blisters and make sure your water bottles are full for tomorrow." As we moved higher on the mountain, we grew to appreciate this level of service even more.

Mary, Claudia B-S and I found a circle of rocks left intact by a previous climbing party and laid out our ground pads and sleeping bags inside it. We invited Jeannie Morris to join us. Annette and Laura teamed up in another circle of rocks, with Vicki and Nancy Knoble close by. Dr. Bud, Paul, Steve and Jimmy found their own circle. The guides—Peter, John, Kurt, Catie, Heather and Jeff—hunkered down together. We were already beginning the process of natural selection, splitting out into tent teams that we would retain on the mountain, although we all would be tentless that night.

Camp was organized by seven o'clock. The sun had dropped behind the ridge above us, but the sky was still bright and the air balmy, about sixty-five degrees. All the mules and the gauchos' horses had maneuvered themselves away from camp, in search of grass.

We noticed that many of the mules had saddle sores. Silvia Quiroga, an Argentine park ranger who was accompanying us to base camp, explained that the sores were caused by the mules being used so much over the past several days. That week alone, three-hundred-and-eighty permits had been issued for the popular Ruta Normal. Permits are issued to each climber, regardless of the size of the climbing party. Only twenty-two permits had been issued for our route, the one leading to base camp at Plaza Argentinas. We didn't expect much company.

By dusk, our camp at Las Lenas was a festive but peaceful site, decorated with purple sleeping bags, green gear duffels and strands of colorful prayer flags stretched across each encampment. Donors to the expedition's fundraising goal had purchased prayer flags in honor of friends and relatives with breast cancer. The names of these friends and relatives had been emblazoned on the flags, and now Expedition Inspiration would carry them to the mountain to honor all women with breast cancer. The prayer flags fluttered in the light breeze and our emotions fluttered with them.

After Vicki returned from her bath in the river, she visited our rock circle. "It was real interesting," she said. "I was with three other women on the team and all three of them have had lumpectomies. The last time I was in a hot desert environment like this was a year-and-a-half ago in the Grand Canyon when I still had two breasts. We all ran around naked and lay on the rocks like lizards, which felt like a very natural thing to do. We were all two-breasted. So it was a first moment for me to be out there today with women who are survivors, like me, but they are still different because they still have their feminine shape and voluptuousness. They asked me why I chose to have a mastectomy. I told them that, first of all, I had had *in situ* cancer which was thought to be pretty extensive. And, also, I didn't want to have radiation.

"Also, I thought if I got cancer again in my breast, I would feel as if I had made a bad decision to keep it. I'd much rather be free and clear of the cancer and have it gone. And if I have a recurrence, radiation will probably be my only weapon to get rid of any cancer that could be in my lungs or my bones. I feel as if I've kept my body clear of radiation so I can use it if the cancer ever comes back."

Being with two-breasted women made her reconsider having reconstruction, Vicki said. "I waffle back and forth because it's just so nice to see two breasts. It'll be different when the rest of the team shows up and there are more mastectomies." She laughed. "Then the one-breasted women will have their own little club and I'll feel totally at home."

Mary reminded Vicki that she and Claudia B-S also had mastectomies and that they were proud to have Vicki as one of them. Then Mary changed the subject. "I'm so glad to finally be on the trail!"

Vicki agreed. "I keep pinching myself. I've been anticipating this for so long, I don't want to miss any moment of it. Seeing the prayer flags with all their colors waving is very moving. I start to cry when I look at them."

That night, we all fell asleep under a billion bright stars with a gentle breeze scudding over the top of our safe enclosures.

The second day of the trek was longer and more grueling, but we got off to an invigorating start with our first river crossing. At Las Lenas, the river runs deeper and faster than in other places, so we enlisted the help of two of the gauchos. Each rode his horse and led a mule across the river with one of us perched aboard. We wore our packs with the waist belts unbuckled. In this way, if we fell in the river, we'd be easier to retrieve without a pack to hinder us. The horses and mules were sure-footed and we suffered no mishaps. Not one to disappoint the photographers, Laura let loose with a "Yee-haw!" as her mount splashed across the river.

We started trekking in shade, but within an hour the sun had risen above the canyon walls and was beating down on us. We lunched at a spot where the valley flattened and the river ran shallow. We took off our boots and soaked our feet in the cold water. The brisk, arid wind that arrived again at noon provided some relief from the heat, but our feet still felt hammered by the time we traveled the eleven miles of extremely rocky terrain between Las Lenas and Casa De Piedras. About a half hour out of Casa de Piedras we were rewarded for our hardships with an incredibly stunning view of Aconcagua, framed by a gap in the canyon wall.

From this vantage point, we could see a good portion of our route on the upper mountain, including where our high camp at 19,000 feet would be situated, and where we would traverse across the Polish Glacier to intersect the Ruta Normal at 20,500 feet. The summit knob wasn't visible, but the mountain, with its fresh mantle of snow, looked sufficiently imposing and beautiful. The team gazed in silence for a few moments, then Laura's "Whoop!" of joy jolted us back into the present moment. We practically floated into camp from there.

We set up tents to provide relief from the wind and dust. We had brand-new, four-season mountaineering tents from JanSport, with our team logo imprinted on the outside of each rain fly. Peter encouraged all of us to practice setting up our tents. "When we get to high camp, it's likely to be cold and windy," he said. "You'll be tired and oxygen-starved and won't want to waste any time getting inside your tent."

The team broke into pairs, many of us choosing to tent with the same partners we had on Rainier: Mary and Jeannie; Laura and Annette; Vicki and Nancy Knoble; Claudia B-S and me; Dr. Bud and Paul; and Jimmy Kay and Steve Marts. The guides split up in pairs: Peter and Kurt; John and Jeff; and Catie and Heather.

After camp was set up, the guides brewed hot drinks and Peter gathered us around to recap the day and talk about the future. Although Laura remained our leader in spirit, Peter took over the reins for the duration of the climb. Before we began the trek to base camp, he told Laura, "I want you to concentrate on staying well and getting up the mountain." Laura had come down with a case of dysentery that Dr. Bud had been treating since we left Los Angeles. As word of her condition spread among the team members, we couldn't help but wonder what would happen if Laura became too ill to climb. Luckily, that question never had to be addressed. The condition cleared up before we left Puenta del Inca. Laura's resiliency and strength were impressive.

To his circle of climbers, Peter announced, "I'd like to propose a toast to a very successful day. You all did a great job, so let's drink to that." We raised our water bottles and drank.

"We're here at the right time," Peter informed us. "This is the most snow I've ever seen on the mountain. All of the storms from a week or so ago are going to really benefit us. The snow should consolidate and give us good walking. We're at about 11,000 feet tonight and we've made the move to this camp pretty comfortably. Tomorrow we're moving up about three thousand feet to base camp. What did you think of the pace yesterday and today?"

Most of us nodded. Someone said, "Great."

"Yesterday and today were just a little faster than what everyone might be comfortable with," said Peter. "There's a reason why we did that. These are trekking days. The climb is going to get rougher as we go up higher. We're going to rest at base camp. And we're going to take a rest day at Camp 1 at 16,000. Even so, we're probably going to be a little beat up when we get on top. You survivors are so good at dealing with discomfort, much more than the average person, and that's going to work in your favor."

Peter offered us encouragement. "That positive mental attitude—PMA—and enthusiasm are wonderful. Keep drawing off that. Sometimes during the trek maybe you're thinking, 'God, it's hot, when is that next break? Boy, I'm thirsty.' Try not to let any of these conditions drag you down. Look around. Look at all these wonderful people with you. This wonderful project. PMA is a good thing to focus on when the going gets tough."

Laura added, "All we have to think about is that we're alive. That's always a boost."

"Exactly," said Peter. "Tomorrow I'd like us to be walking by nine o'clock. It's going to take a little longer, with the tents, to break camp. You all did great this morning; everything went smoothly. It took less than seven hours to get here. A realistic time tomorrow also would be about seven hours. We only have nine miles to go, but most of it is up. I'm going to ask that no one play Walkmans for the first couple hours."

He turned and pointed across the floor of the valley to a notch in the canyon. "You can see the Relinchos Valley river gorge and the Relinchos River. This is a sharply defined gorge. I've seen some good-sized rocks come down in there. So we need to be listening through this first stretch. You'll notice that the guides will be on alert. We won't take any long breaks. We want to move through quickly and not expose ourselves to objective hazards."

The Relinchos River was fed by glacial melt off Aconcagua. "After a couple of hours, we'll emerge from the gorge and reach a large moraine," Peter explained. "From the top of that we'll be able to see the mountain. From there on, you can break out the Walkmans.

"We'll also have a few river crossings tomorrow, so throw your sandals or river-crossing shoes into your pack. With so much snow on the mountain, the crossings could be, shall we say, a little more exciting than what we've already experienced. But that's the beauty of climbing. You never know what you're going to encounter or how the weather will behave. Bring single-layer gloves and long pants. It will be warm when we start out, but we usually end up changing into long pants before we reach base camp. If there's any wind up there, it'll be cold. Bring your fleece jackets, too.

"The moraine is steep in several areas, so we'll get a good workout," Peter added. "We'll slow down the pace and start blowing a few pressure breaths, breathing a little harder. We've had three nights at 9,000 feet and tonight we're sleeping at 11,000 feet. Tomorrow we're moving up to 13,800. In terms of acclimatization, this is ideal. Three days of good workout followed by a rest, and we'll be right on line. So what's the number one priority here on Expedition Inspiration?"

In unison we replied, "Safety!"

"That's right. We all have important things to do after this trip. We want to continue living our lives. What's the second priority?"

"Summit!"

"Summit, you bet. We've got to get it and I think we will. And the third?"

"Fun!"

"Yes, although with this group," said Peter, "fun is really right up there with priorities one and two. Many of you have slept at 14,000 feet; some have slept at higher altitudes. A few of you haven't slept higher than 10,000 feet. Fourteen thousand feet is above the level where things grow. The human body is amazing. We can adjust—if we take the time, drink lots of fluids and be smart in taking care of ourselves. After we adjust to 14,000 feet, we'll work our way to Camp 1 at 16,200. We'll carry a load up there, dump it, then come back down to sleep at base camp. Then we'll move up to 16,200 and sleep. We'll follow the same routine to move to Camp 2 at 19,000 feet. 'Carry high, sleep low.' That's the best way to acclimatize. We guides will keep an eye on you and trust you to be open and honest. Tell us if you're having a problem. Our goal is to get everyone to the top of this mountain—but we won't compromise safety."

After Peter's talk, I asked Laura, "What's been your best moment so far?"

"The first step," she said. "Getting started. So much has gone into this project and to actually be moving toward our goal in honor of all women is so exciting. I'm real pleased that Peter picked this mountain. What an incredible trek in. The mountain is fabulous. It's the most beautiful mountain I've ever seen. Everybody's healthy. This trip couldn't be more perfect."

A party of five men came into our camp after dinner and introduced themselves. They were from the U.S. and knew Peter and Kurt. They had heard of Expedition Inspiration and had summited Aconcagua two days before. They reported that the weather had been decent and the route was in terrific condition. Also, they told us, any snow that may have been in base camp or at Camp 1 had all either melted or been blown away. We were relieved to hear this news. Base camp would be easier to establish on rock. Snow makes an uneven platform when melting out from under a tent full of warm bodies.

As the sky dimmed and the air grew cold, we retreated to our tents. Annette came by to show me and Claudia B-S a gift she had received from the gauchos. She and Laura had presented them with commemorative Expedition Inspiration hats. "I also took some pictures of them and one of them gave me his *faja*," Annette said, holding up a colorful woven band. "It's a wraparound belt. It's beautiful, don't you think?"

"The first condor sighting and now the belt. You're lucky."

"They told me that the condor is the king of the Andes, like the lion is the king of the jungle." Annette paused for a moment, took a deep breath and continued. "You know, I can't remember being any happier or more at peace than I am now. The whole trip in has made me very happy. I felt like dancing most of the day today. I feel so great, so strong and excited about being here."

Peter interrupted us to ask Annette to accompany him back to the gauchos' camp, to translate plans for tomorrow's move to base camp. Annette had grown up in Venezuela, and her fluent Spanish had been much in demand during the trip. "Don't let him trade women for mules," we called after Annette as she left with Peter.

After the negotiations, Annette returned to our tent. She said, "Wasn't last night awesome? From the beginning, I'd been looking forward to sleeping outside under the stars. They are more beautiful than I had imagined. And then hearing something I hadn't imagined: the prayer flags blowing in the wind. What energy! I could visualize all the prayers going up in the air with the prayer flags. I'm so glad we have them with us."

Annette spied the bag of snacks that Claudia B–S had stashed by her sleeping bag. "I have apricots, apples, peaches, nuts and candy," said Claudia as she handed the bag to Annette. "Jim went to the store for me. He knows how hungry I get. I was on McKinley in 1983 and I ran out of snacks on my first day, at 15,000 feet. We still had to camp at 18,000."

"To me, running out of food is a nightmare," Annette agreed.

We took our pulses. Mine was eighty, Annette's was eighty-eight and Claudia's was one hundred. "We're pumped!" exclaimed Annette.

"Claudia has been stuffing salt into her body with all those peanuts. That's why her pulse is so high."

Vicki stuck her head in the tent. "We're the luckiest ladies on earth at this moment," she pronounced.

"No kidding," said Annette. "We don't have to be indoors for three weeks."

Annette bade us good-night and Vicki crawled in to talk. She helped herself to some dried apricots. "I think we'll all make it to 19,000 feet, at least to the carry," Vicki speculated.

"Why are you mentally stopping there?" I asked.

"Because most of us haven't been to that altitude. I haven't, anyway. It will be interesting. Claudia, you said you felt awful on McKinley, right?"

"At 18,000 feet you can't even tie your boots. Your movements become slow and methodical. You only carry up what you need. I had a headache that started at 16,000 and stayed with me. You get used to it."

After Vicki said good-night, Claudia lay back on her bag and said, "I really have changed my thinking about all this since Mount Rainier. It's been a year since my diagnosis and I'm now totally healthy. And I realize for me to be healthy, I have to get away from having been a cancer patient. When I first came into the group, I was still in chemotherapy. I hadn't had the chance to talk to people or to a support group. Since I finished chemotherapy last August, I've taken a close look at my illness and I've asked myself how I might have benefited from being sick. For one thing, I got out of a stressful situation at school.

"I began taking time every day to examine what type of stress might be present and see what I could do about it. By November, I felt a real difference. The effects of chemo were gone, I was back in my full running and workout routine, I felt free of stress. I had never stopped running, but I'd had to slow down a bit during my treatments. It's hard when the team gets together for a TV or newspaper interview to keep telling my story of illness over again. I think as we keep going back to our stories of cancer, we get something from repeating them, and I'm afraid we might never get away from the experience. And that might lead to a recurrence. I don't know. Who knows? All I do know is, to be well, I need to focus on right now, on my wellness. To me, this climb is a celebration of *wellness.*"

The usually laconic Claudia B–S ended her story with her trademark grin and crawled out of the tent for one last look at the stars.

My last thoughts before sleep were of home and the trek team. Today, they had left Los Angeles for Buenos Aires. If all went as planned, they would arrive in base camp as we made our move to high camp at 19,000 feet. From a logistical standpoint, bringing in the two teams separately made sense. On the other hand, when we gathered for meals or to discuss our progress or to hang our prayer flags, the absence of our other teammates was poignantly noticed. Our bond had been forged on the flanks of Mount Rainier and reinforced in the mountains of Sun Valley during our last full team meeting. Here in Argentina, with our goal looming nearer each day, that bond was becoming stronger than ever.

Thursday, January 26, dawned as another beautiful day, a "summit day," in Peter's words. We worried that we would use up too many summit days before the real one arrived. How long could this perfect weather last? Argentina was having its summer but we were at the foot of the highest mountain in the Western Hemisphere, a mountain that made its own weather. A week ago, Aconcagua had conjured up a storm that dumped more snow than the Argentine park rangers had seen in twenty summers.

To spend time worrying about the weather was futile at this point. As Peter had reminded us in Puenta del Inca, we were prepared for anything. And we were determined to reach our goal. Bursting with energy, we packed up camp by eight-fifteen, nearly an hour ahead of schedule. Peter was delighted. We were excited. By the end of the day, we would be in base camp, the symbolic beginning point of all expeditions. From that camp, we would stage our assault on Aconcagua, and continue the symbolic assault on breast cancer.

The sun hadn't yet popped above the canyon wall and the morning air was cool. To get to the Relinchos Valley, we had to cross the Río de Las Vacas once more. Here the river had divided into three narrow but deep fingers of rushing water. We enlisted the help of our gauchos to once again ferry us across in style.

The trail through the gorge of the Relinchos Valley was rocky, narrow and steep. We had to cross the river in three places. In two spots, the guides strung a rope across the river for us to hold onto as we jumped from one boulder to another to get to the other side. The third crossing was narrow and shallow enough to navigate barefoot. The cold water was soothing to our aching, blistered feet.

We worked hard all day. Peter slowed the pace as we advanced into higher altitude. To conserve energy, we began rest-stepping and pressure breathing. At the top of the gorge, the moraine flattened out and gave us an awe-inspiring view of the snow-covered upper mountain.

At four o'clock, we marched into base camp. We whooped, hollered and hugged, and then sat down on our packs for a ten minute break, reveling in the sight of this beautiful mountain. There was no snow at base camp nor most of the way up to 16,200-foot Camp 1.

A stiff breeze had come up but the sky was sunny and clear. The terrain was as expected: rocky. Many previous expeditions had cleared tent sites. We hauled our gear, all fifty-seven duffels, to various sites, with Peter shouting gleefully, "Great training for the upper mountain! Don't you love it?"

Everyone was feeling the jump in altitude from 11,000 to 13,800. Setting up our tent seemed to take Claudia B-S and me forever. We frequently ran out of energy and had to stop and take deep breaths. As soon as the tent was erected, I threw in my ground pad and sleeping bag and stretched out for a half hour.

Ever energetic, Claudia B-S busied herself by organizing her gear. Eventually, we had everything with us inside the tent, arranged in stuff sacks or piles, including our precious bags of snacks. When the sun dipped behind the peaks surrounding base camp, we changed into thermal underwear for the first time on the trek.

Claudia B-S took off her socks and immediately stuck her feet out the tent door. "Hoowee! Guess I'll have to wash these suckers tomorrow. It's Baby Wipe time."

One of our hygienic routines in camp was to wipe our hands with Baby Wipes before meals. Peter provided the wipes as part of the group gear. Several of us had also brought individual stashes of wipes, for those times when a river wasn't handy. After three days on the trail, this was one of those times.

During our dinner of rice, chili and fresh oranges that night, we all commented about how the mountain looked much more beautiful than we had imagined after watching Peter's slide show a few months ago. Now, with the mantle of snow on the upper mountain and the striking gradients of red and gray stone on its lower flanks, Mount Aconcagua seemed the most beautiful place on earth.

Peter announced that our plan for tomorrow, Friday, January 27, was to take the day off. We'd hang around base camp, reinforce some rock walls, wash laundry in a nearby stream. We had brought several Solar Showers, rubberized plastic bags with hoses that serve as showers in the wilderness. Fill with water in the morning, let hang in the sun for a few hours, *et voilà*! You have a warm shower.

By eight-thirty that night, the wind had come up and we had retired to our tents. Claudia B-S celebrated our arrival in base camp by eating a bedtime Snickers. We read and listened to sounds—mostly giggles—from the other tents. At dinner, everyone was cheerful; no one was suffering from any ill effects of altitude.

~

Nature called me out of the tent just before Friday's sunrise and treated me to a rare sight: the crescent moon with Venus at its lower tip, shining in the morning sky. I thought of home, where I knew my friend Francey, who had supported me in my training for the climb, would be looking at the same sight. Not a cloud in sight, not a breath of wind. Another beautiful day was dawning—another summit day.

Later that morning, walking through base camp, I stopped to talk to two climbers who had summited two days before. They had taken the same route we planned to follow. They said that the route was in good shape and that the "dreaded Canaleta," a steep, scree-and-boulder-filled chute immediately below the summit, was lined with snow, which made for easier walking. However, they added, that snow was melting quickly.

One of the climbers was a woman named Ann from Connecticut. Her guide was Jim Williams, a well-known professional guide from the Northeast. Ann had read about Expedition Inspiration in *Women's Sports & Fitness*, and was excited to be on the mountain at the same time as we. She walked over to our camp to meet the rest of the team. When she first arrived in base camp, she said the area had been covered in snow and storms had swept through every afternoon. We took her photo with the team and gave her a team T-shirt.

Next, two men came over to visit. They said that they had been climbing on Rainier last July at the same time we were on our shakedown climb. They had bought team shirts in their home towns. They also had their pictures taken with the team. Seeing both men and women share enthusiasm for our cause was extremely gratifying.

At breakfast Peter announced that we'd be spending an extra

day in base camp to further acclimatize. We all felt great but the weather seemed to be in a holding pattern. Peter wanted us to be as accustomed to the altitude as possible.

"Every day, my admiration grows for each of you," Peter told the team. "With mountaineering, you have the choice of being here. When you got cancer, you had no choice. You were basically dealt a hand and didn't have a choice of whether or not to follow that course. But you survived. The goal of mountaineering is also to survive, to make a round trip of the adventure. Sometimes the survival involves the summit, and sometimes it doesn't. The survivors have told us how their experience with breast cancer brought them close to the edge and added new meaning to their lives. The same thing happens in mountaineering. Living close to the edge makes you feel more alive. That's why we choose to be here."

During the trek to base camp, each of the survivors seemed intensely appreciative of every moment, whether it included an incredible sunrise or the brilliant stars, the expanse of clear sky, the river crossings, the challenging rocky gorges, the condor sightings, the interactions with the gauchos and other climbers. Everything was a delight and a discovery. We joked a lot, but the underlying feeling was that life is precious; it's good to be alive. The survivors' attitudes had been inspiring to those of us on the support team. The survivors had taken to calling us the "nonsurvivors," an ominous appellation at best.

Peter's idea of a rest day at base camp meant building more tent sites and excavating two platforms, a large one for the dining tent and a smaller one below to serve as a patio. The platforms were separated by a rock retaining wall. Peter divided us into "feeders," "builders" and "scratchers." The feeders brought rocks to the builders while the scratchers cleared away the surplus of dirt and rock to help flatten the surface for the builders.

"Working like this, down here at this elevation," said Peter, "is like putting money in the bank."

Peter decided to increase our investment by also building a shitter. It would be more environmentally friendly for eighteen people to poop in the same hole rather than under or on any available rock—a practice that, judging by the amount of dried excrement and soiled paper littering base camp, had been popular until our arrival. We dug a deep hole, topped it with large, flat rocks appropriate for squatting, and constructed a chest-high, three-sided wall of rocks for privacy. Other climbing parties watched us labor from a distance and, by the next day, they had started using the new privy, too.

Annette christened the latrine. Afterwards, she announced that it had been her "first time outdoors." We all offered our congratulations. She explained that Claudia B-S had coached her. "Claudia told me all I needed was a rock to lean on and a good view," said Annette. "I'm here to tell you: the view from our privy at base camp beats the hell out of any magazine."

With the construction finished, Peter gave us the rest of the day off. Most of us read, wrote in journals and talked. Not Claudia B-S. She recruited John for a game of Nerf football. Activity was her way of unwinding from physical exertion. We watched her running for passes and laughing, laughing, laughing. Not one of us had a doubt that Claudia B-S would stand on the summit of Aconcagua. She was strong and had an incredible, infectious, positive spirit.

Neither did we doubt that Laura would also reach her goal. During "Expedition Excavation" that morning, Laura stated that the first time she ever understood how the Egyptians had built the pyramids was during her seven weeks in the hospital isolation tent for intensive chemotherapy. "There I had such a singular focus," she reflected. "I realized that if you focus all your energy solely on one goal, you can do anything—build pyramids, climb mountains, get well."

That afternoon, Dr. Bud commented on the value of Laura's incredible resiliency as an example for others. "Yesterday, while we were trekking to base camp, I was thinking about how unbelievable it was to watch a bone marrow transplant walk up this mountain. As a physician, I know how debilitating that treatment can be to someone who survives it. In Laura's case, high dose chemotherapy followed by a bone marrow transplant, complicated by pneumonia and lymphedema, both of which she overcame—and five years later I'm watching her walk up this mountain. It's unbelievable."

He added, "The value of what we're seeing here has such a broad scope. It's not that every person who has chemotherapy or a bone marrow transplant or significant medical care followed by severe side effects is going to climb a 23,000-foot mountain. And it's not that some people aren't going to get sick with those treatments. But it does show the range of what is possible. It shows what the human will and spirit can do. If it's possible for one or five or ten people, then it's possible for more.

"It's also a great example for physicians that they can present to patients. Not to say, 'Don't worry about chemotherapy, nothing will happen, you'll be able to climb a mountain afterward.' That's not the message. The message is that people can overcome great afflictions."

That same day, after a lunch of tuna sandwiches, chicken noodle soup and fresh apples, the team got into a discussion about whether or not to wear underwear to the summit. They seemed to be fairly evenly divided on the matter. In fact, tentmates were also much in alignment. Peter listened to the discussion and then commented that perhaps we had not expended enough energy that morning. He suggested a walk that led over a flat part of the moraine to the head of a valley adjacent to base camp. Claudia B–S was the only one who took him up on the suggestion. When she returned, she announced, "I walked to the end of the valley, right below the peaks at snow level. Found a snow melt creek with a great pool. I stripped off my clothes, washed my underwear and my socks, washed me and then lay out on a rock in the sun while my clothes dried. I am rejuvenated!"

Later, in Vicki and Nancy Knoble's tent, there was some serious reflection. Nancy Knoble told me, "This is a place I would have never dreamed of being. It's not something that I would have put on my life list of personal goals, to be on an expedition on Aconcagua. It's beyond that. It's already one of the most incredible experiences I've ever had. Getting here to base camp makes it real. To me, being on a summit of a mountain is very spiritual. It's exciting, wonderful, enriching."

She continued: "When I was first asked to be on the expedition, one of the things I thought I could do would be to dedicate the climb to a few other people so that I'd feel as if I had my own personal team going up with me. So I've dedicated my climb to three friends who had breast cancer before me: Cathie, Becky and Sharon—and to Francine, my radiation oncologist, who has become one of the dearest people in my life. When I get to the summit, it will be for them, not solely for me.

"As we went through the fundraising process before the climb, we met hundreds and hundreds of people. What really impressed me was how people connected with this climb and the concept behind it. And how they really have felt a part of it by contributing in some way. All the people wearing Expedition

Inspiration T-shirts and sweatshirts are going to feel every bit as excited about the summit as we will when we get up there because they've invested a part of themselves in this project. It's also interesting how many people have told me that they, too, have breast cancer, or that their mom, daughter, sister or friend was recently diagnosed. You can hardly be in a group of three or four people and not find someone who has had a close, recent experience with breast cancer.

"For me, the important message from this expedition is awareness. It's vital that women be aware. I have met so many women who say, 'I don't have it in my family. I don't have to worry about this. It's not going to happen to me.' They're not doing self-exams, they're over forty and not getting mammograms on a regular basis. They're putting their heads in the sand. It's helpful to be able to explain to them that ninety percent of women who get breast cancer don't have it in their families. The expedition helps all of us share our stories, which cause people to realize, 'She's like me. That could happen to me.'"

Vicki asked, rhetorically, "When we get to the summit, are we going to have any energy left to cry? When I walked into base camp, it hit me. My God, all these months of working out and working for the climb and now here we are. Coming up the Relinchos Valley, I kept waiting to get above the vegetation line because I knew that base camp had to be above that. And then finally we were here. It kind of looks like the dark side of the moon."

Vicki added, "A couple of weeks ago, I realized that this has been a real healing process for me. I got my cancer in October a year ago, and applied for the team while undergoing chemo. I was accepted in April and then I didn't finish chemo until June. The following six months were filled with Rainier, local fundraising events, newspaper and TV interviews, working out. It was a quick six months compared to the six months of chemo that seemed to pass slowly. I realize now that it's all connected: diagnosis, surgery, chemo, working out, fundraising, the expedition. I think I'm coming full circle into a bigger healing picture. I felt I made a major summit, going through chemo. That was one of the hardest summits I've ever had to make. There were times I wanted to turn back, didn't want to finish. If I can stand on top of Aconcagua, I think that I will probably feel the most alive I've ever felt in my life."

Although all of us on the team had tear-filled moments, humor was our constant companion. At one point, Laura said, "We're happy to be alive. I have a sign on my kitchen wall that says, 'A day in which you have not laughed is the most wasted day of all.'"

"I tried to make the best of my surgery and treatment," Mary said, and proceeded to tell the group about the smiley face that her daughter had drawn on Mary's breast before surgery.

"What happened when your doctor saw it?"

"I really don't know. I remember the nurse did suggest that we wipe it off, but I was adamant—it had to stay on. After I awoke from surgery, I forgot about it."

We agreed that Mary's story was funny, although a little unnerving. "I have this vision of that smiley-face breast sitting in a stainless steel bowl," said Laura. "To have humor at that point is extraordinary."

On a lighter note, Laura added, "After I lost all the hair on my body, I came out of the shower one morning and said to Roger, 'This gives *naked* a whole new meaning.'"

Jeannie asked Laura about her anxiety level here at base camp. "In Puenta del Inca, when we heard about the storm, there were a few moments when I thought that this could turn out to be a whole lot worse that we expected," Laura said. "You never know what is going to happen. Now we're at base camp, everybody's healthy, the weather's looking good. What I'm feeling is a good, nervous excitement. This will be the biggest challenge any of us has undergone, short of living through breast cancer."

Before the summit team moved to 16,200 feet to establish Camp 1, we gathered for what would be our last full circle together. We shared the talismans and good-luck treasures that other breast cancer sufferers or families and friends had sent along to inspire and protect us during the climb.

Claudia B-S brought a guardian angel from a close friend in her hometown of Fernley, Nevada, and a book of meditations from another friend, Connie, who had a double mastectomy the year before. Connie had chosen not to have chemotherapy because, as Claudia explained with a grim look on her usually cheerful face, "She doesn't have insurance."

Vicki brought a scarf full of signatures from a fundraising concert she had held in Santa Cruz. She also carried photos of her children, Katy and Jonathan, and a small ice-ax pin from Lou Whittaker. She, too, had a guardian angel that her daughter had bought for her in the airport gift shop. Larry, who had become her workout partner, had given her an owl feather.

Mary held up a T-shirt that had been signed by everyone she worked with at L.L. Bean. On the back of the shirt was embroidered, "There's no woman like a Yeo-woman." She also carried a prayer flag for one of her coworkers who had died of breast cancer the previous spring. "I have a wonderful family," Mary said, as she started to cry. "Five daughters and two sons. I'm taking myself up the mountain because I don't want my daughters to go through what I went through."

Laura's most prized possession was a medicine bag that her

younger sister, Lisa, had made for her. It contained many items, among them a photo of her dog, Buster, a guardian angel and a card from Roger that read, "Just because you're you, I love you." She was also carrying a prayer flag for a friend, Susan McGuire, who had lost the fight against breast cancer a few months ago. There was a Saint Christopher medal from her grandmother, and a tiny fox figurine from her friend Mary Brent. Laura said, "When I was in the hospital, Mary came every single night, and whether I was asleep or awake, put her arms through the plastic sleeves and held my hand. I'm carrying her good spirit for all of us."

Annette also had a medicine bag that she said was "full of energy and support from a lot of different sources." These sources included thirty women in Seattle who had formed a breast cancer support group. Each woman had chosen a day from the trek and dedicated that day of her life to doing something positive about breast cancer, such as accompanying another woman to chemo, visiting surgery patients, participating in fundraising activities or sending energy to the team members. Annette also carried prayer flags for each of these women. Another source was Lisa McGovern, who would pull her family together every night of the climb and do a dance in the team's honor. The third-grade class of Garrison Forest School, of which Annette's goddaughter, Annie, was a member, also had formed a support group. "They have assured me that there's enough energy in here for all of us," said Annette.

I, too, carried a guardian angel from friends and a "Bliss Angel" that another lifelong friend had made for me. Other friends had given me a medallion of Saint Bernard, the patron saint of skiers and alpinists. My partner Francey had sent along a note that I could carry to the summit. In part, it read, "Enclosed are my warm, concentrated thoughts and energy to assist your every step, breath and drink of refreshing water."

A rabbi who was a client of Dr. Bud advised him to "pray as if everything depends on God, but act as if everything depends on you," and gave Bud a talisman from the "miracle rabbi in Jerusalem" to take to the summit. On the back was a prayer from the Old Testament for people going on a long journey.

Holding up a toy biplane, Paul said, "It got pretty dicey before we were to leave on this journey, because a week before Christmas, my father-in-law died. Bob was a good friend—and a pilot, so I'm taking this biplane to the top for Bob and then I'm giving it to his wife, Connie."

Nancy Knoble had the largest array of talismans from and in honor of various friends and family members. Most interesting and touching was a small vial. "These are some of my father's ashes," Nancy explained. "He died two years ago. He was my best friend. He got me interested in the outdoors and took me camping from the age of two. I took a little bit of him to the top of Mount Elbrus and I'll take a little bit of him to the top of each peak I climb so that he can share in my adventures."

Afterward, Laura shared some of her concerns. "What if somebody gets hurt? What if somebody uses up their energy early on? These thoughts come to me and I know others are thinking them." We all nodded, our attention riveted on Laura. This was the first time that she had spoken of anything remotely connected to failure to meet our goal.

"I think what we have to do is look at this as a climb," she continued. "I personally have to stay as fit as I can and keep my mind centered and not start thinking about all the people at home that we'll let down if we don't make it. If there are times when thinking about those people helps you gather more inner strength, then fine. But, I think, basically, we have to say, 'We're here to climb this mountain and we're going to do it. We're going to give ourselves the best opportunity we can.'"

Heather, one of the guides supporting the camera team, spoke up. "I think you all should realize that you have already made a difference. The woman who just walked out of her doctor's office after being diagnosed with breast cancer doesn't care if you make it to 23,000 feet or not. It's enough that you're here. It's the journey—and that's what life and climbing are all about."

As in life, the journey of climbing a mountain can also involve obstacles, setbacks and disappointments. Mount Aconcagua was indifferent to all our charms, talismans, well-wishers and noble intentions, and forced us to struggle for every step we gained from base camp on up. Dr. Bud's rabbi was right: we had to proceed as though everything depended on us. The mountain would not give an inch.

On Sunday, January 29, it took the summit team eight hours to carry half its gear and food from 13,800-foot base camp to 16,200-foot Camp 1, stow it there in stuff sacks anchored by large rocks and return to base camp to sleep for one more night. The weather had been clear and crisp, although Peter had noted high cirrus clouds "and other stuff floating around." One of the Argentine rangers at base camp had told him that a weather report from Chile forecast a storm during the next four days. Peter told us, "It doesn't matter—we're moving to Camp 1, even in marginal weather. Our food and warm clothing are already up there. That's where we want to be."

Peter heard no argument from the team. We were anxious to move closer to the summit also.

That evening, Peter was able to exchange a sporadic radio transmission with Tuck and Erika at Puenta del Inca. The trek team had arrived safely and was gearing up for the hike to base camp. The news was heartening. By Thursday, February 2, they would be in base camp and the entire Expedition Inspiration

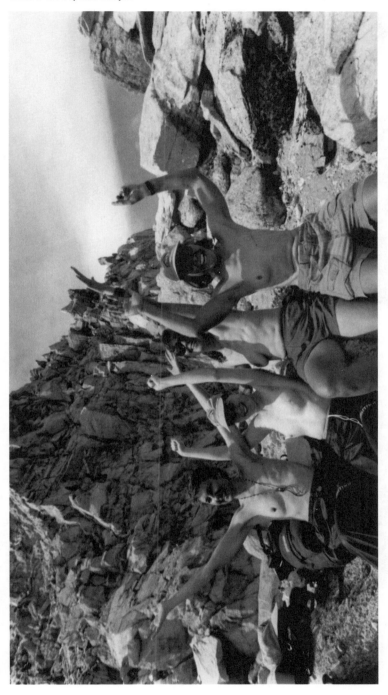

Celebrating wellness on a training climb, Matterhorn Peak, California. Left to right: Sue Anne Foster, Roberta Fama, Vicki Boriack, Claudia Berryman-Shafer.

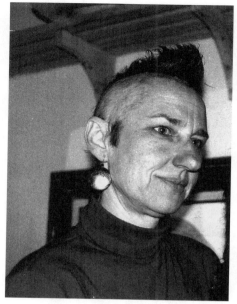

"Mom tried to keep her sense of humor by letting my sister and me shave her hair into a mohawk."
— Mignon Foster, daughter of Sue Anne

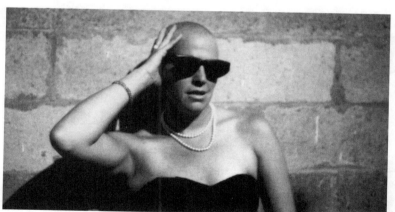

"It doesn't have to be with a hat and a wig and a scarf. It can be bald. It can be okay."
— Annette Porter

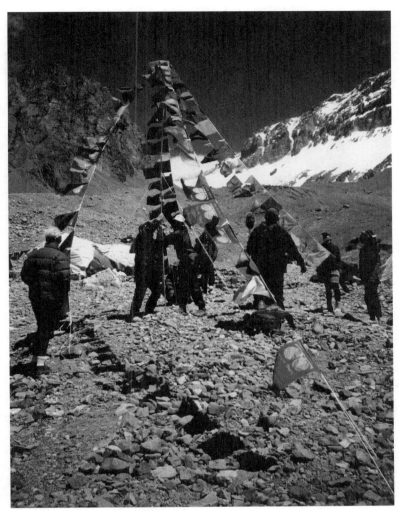

Prayer flag ceremony, Aconcagua base camp.

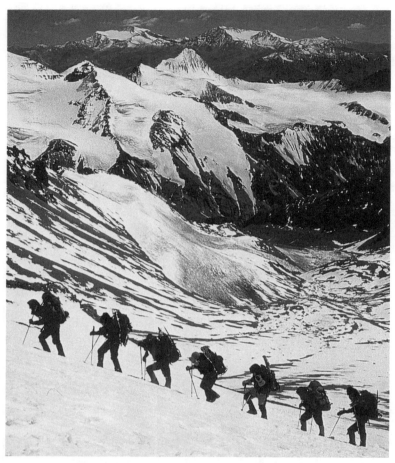

Summit team at 18,000, on the way to Camp 2.

Summit and trek teams at their first glimpse of Aconcagua, outside Puenta del Inca.

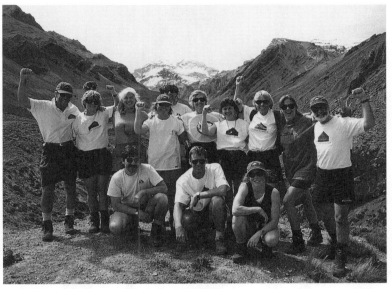

Summit team, bottom row, left to right: John Hanron, Kurt Wedburg, Catie Casson.
Top row: Dr. Bud Alpert, Andrea Gabbard, Nancy Knoble, Claudia Berryman-Shafer,
Peter Whittaker, Mary Yeo, Vicki Boriack, Laura Evans, Annette Porter, Paul Delorey.

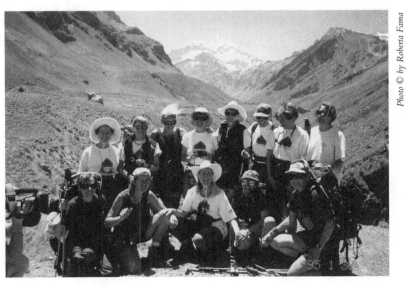

Trek team, bottom row, left to right: Sue Anne Foster, Nancy Hudson, Roberta Fama,
Andrea Martin, Dr. Kathleen Grant. Top row: Sara Hildebrand, Patty Duke, Saskia
Thiadens, Kim O'Meara Anderson, Claudia Crosetti, Nancy Johnson, Eleanor Davis,
Ashley Sumner-Cox

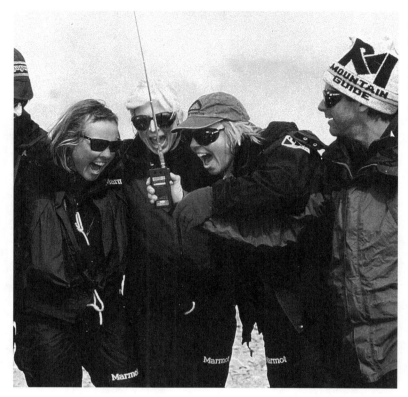

Victory call from the summit: "We're standing up here in honor of all women."
Left to right: Claudia Berryman-Shafer, Nancy Knoble, Laura Evans, Peter Whittaker.

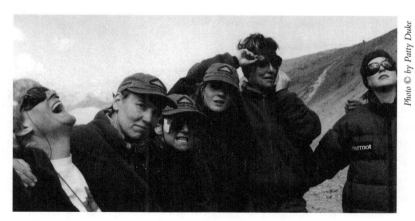

The news reaches base camp. Left to right: Andrea Gabbard, Nancy Johnson, Andrea Martin, Ashley Sumner-Cox, Kim O'Meara Anderson, Roberta Fama.

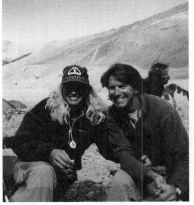

Erika and Peter Whittaker
at base camp.

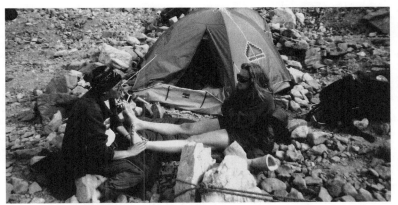

Sue Anne's massage parlor, open for business. Sue Anne gives Annette the treatment.

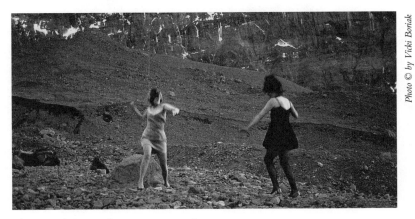

Eleanor and Annette dance up a storm at base camp.

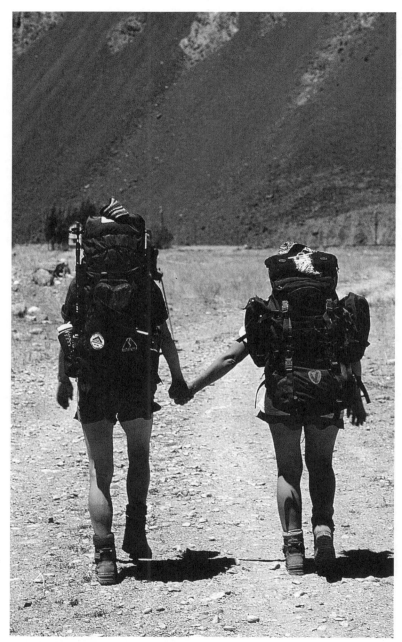

Nancy Knoble and Vicki Boriack, on the way home.

team would be together on the mountain. If all went as planned, Thursday would be the day of our summit bid.

Whoever said, "Life is what happens while you're busy making plans" must have been a mountain climber, or a cancer survivor. On Saturday, we packed the rest of the gear and food we would need for the higher camps. The food alone weighed over a hundred pounds, but was divided into manageable amounts and dispersed among the team. Anything not needed for high camp was left at base camp in the large duffels that the mules had transported. Jeannie stayed in base camp in one of the smaller tents, while Steve advanced with the team. Guides Heather and Jeff carried Steve's extra camera batteries and film cassettes.

Four hours later, all but two team members had reached Camp 1. Mary had fallen behind and Kurt had stayed with her. While they advanced to Camp 1 at a slower pace, we set up tents, dug a new shitter and started building rock walls around our tents to protect them from the wind, which blew stronger and more persistently at this elevation. Since we had fewer tents than at base camp, Mary moved in with Claudia B-S and me. Mary had an L.L. Bean down-insulated sleeping bag with a warmth rating of minus thirty degrees. We put her between us and the effect was that of a heater radiating from the middle of the tent.

Mary, a cheerful, positive person with a degree of good ol' Yankee reserve, had little to say about falling off pace. "I had trouble coordinating pressure breathing and rest-stepping," she said. She also had developed climber's cough, a dry hacking cough that is a side effect of exertion at high altitude. We offered words of understanding and encouragement and then focused our attention on the howling winds outside. That evening at Camp 1, the mountain unleashed the first obstacle, the first test of our endurance. The storm that had been forecast by the Chileans rolled into camp like a freight train. High winds and blowing snow pummeled our tents mercilessly and kept us huddled inside, immobilized, for two days and three nights.

At base camp, Jeannie literally held down the fort, filling her tent with gear, and herself, to keep it attached to the ground. The wind licked and tore at the large base-camp tents, flattening one and mutilating the other.

Undaunted by news of bad weather, the twenty-four members of the trek team prepared to depart Puenta del Inca for base camp, as planned.

Winds of Healing

Before leaving for South America, Nancy Hudson
had spent her last few days at home making "spirit stones" for
each team member. She had gathered a number of small rocks
and painted a different animal on each. When Nancy presented
the stones to the team, she explained that, in Native American
folklore, animals were seen as totems or symbols that played a
crucial role in the wheel of life. Land animals were the protec-
tors. Air creatures embodied spirituality and wisdom. Water
creatures were healers. Each team member selected a stone as
her personal totem to carry on the trek.

Sue Anne carried a large Earth flag to South America. En-
circling the globe on the flag were the names of all the breast
cancer survivors on the team, in gold ink. In the space outside
that area were hundreds of names of other cancer victims, living

and dead. Sue Anne had been carrying the flag everywhere for several months. "It seems that wherever I go, someone either has cancer or knows someone who does," she said. "Students at my daughter's school wrote President Clinton's mother's name, Virginia Kelly, on the flag. People at the supermarket, at the post office—nearly everyone has a name to add."

On the flight to Buenos Aires, the pilot made an announcement in both Spanish and English about Expedition Inspiration and the Earth flag that was to be carried up the mountain. Sue Anne invited anyone on the airplane who had cancer or knew someone with cancer to contribute a name. The flight attendants circulated the flag, and many names were added.

Sue Anne also carried two items that, she said, "were not essential in the guides' eyes." One was a wooden prayer arrow with feathers that she had obtained from a Hopi and Navajo ceremony. The other was a wooden spirit stick. Sue Anne explained, "I attached a few stalks of wheat to the stick, to represent my Kansas birthplace. Other people gave me little trinkets and fetishes to take up the mountain and I attached all of them to the Spirit Stick. It represented the spirit of the trek team." She planned to leave the prayer arrow at base camp after the climb.

During the team's stay in Mendoza, Claudia Crosetti observed in her journal: "Of anyone on the trek team, Sue Anne is the one who really 'lives in the moment.' We had a group meeting last night at six o'clock and Sue Anne didn't show up until eight, when we were getting ready to go out to dinner. Everyone was worried and Tuck was not happy. He reminded us that we needed to stick together. As it turned out, Sue Anne had gone to a local park, met some people who put names on her prayer flag, then went with a couple to a relative's house to get another signature. She never heard the announcement about a team meeting."

On their second and last night in Mendoza, the trek team had dinner at El Meson, a renowned Spanish restaurant where climbers traditionally eat their last decent meal before departing for the mountain. Entertainment is provided by Charlie, a blind piano player who invites the audience to sing along. The entire team stood with arms linked at the piano, swaying and singing to Paul Simon's "Bridge Over Troubled Water."

Claudia Crosetti remarked later that this was the most moving moment of the trip for her. "Dr. Kathleen Grant, my physician, stood with her arm around me while we sang," she said. "I felt such incredible support and love. I realized we were all like a bridge over troubled water, having come full circle through our diseases to this place in Argentina to celebrate our lives together."

The trek team also hiked to the vantage point outside Puenta del Inca for their first glimpse of Aconcagua. They were accompanied by a writer and photographer from *Gente*, Argentina's version of *People* magazine. A feature story on the climb appeared in the magazine while the team was still in Argentina.

After the hike, Eleanor and Sara met a man back in Puenta del Inca who had just returned from summiting Aconcagua. After hearing about the nature of Expedition Inspiration, the climber gave them some sage advice. "Do not be concerned about getting to the top. The summit is in your heart." For the trek team, the summit was certainly a heartfelt goal, if not a physical one.

As the summit team had done before advancing to Camp 1, the trek team gathered in a circle on their last afternoon in Puenta del Inca to share their feelings about the climb. "Most of us talked about how proud we were to be part of such an inspirational undertaking," Claudia Crosetti wrote in her journal. Twenty-one-year-old Ashley revealed that her mother had been recently diagnosed with breast cancer, and added, "I am climbing in her honor." Roberta, who had suffered a recurrence, reminded her team, "If it happens to you, I want you to know that it doesn't mean it's the end."

Guide Ned broke into tears and related how his mother had died of cancer when he was nineteen. "I don't think she was able to fight as hard as all of you have," he said, holding the hands of team members on either side of him.

Dr. Kathleen Grant described the summit team as "the physical part of the team; they are the body. The trek team is the heart." She also described gentle Mark Tucker as "the man who shepherded us up the mountain." Later, she nicknamed Peter "the General" for the way he marched us off the mountain. The two team leaders became forever stuck with their apt and loving monikers: Tuck, the Shepherd; Peter, the General.

Nancy Hudson mentioned that the climb was merely the icing on the cake for her after so many months of training and fundraising in her community. The team had some more "icing" planned for Nancy. That night after dinner, the lights went out in the dining hall and in walked one of the waiters with a brightly lit, homemade birthday cake which Ana, the Argentine park ranger who would accompany the team to base camp, had managed to procure. After singing a boisterous "Happy Birthday," the team gave forty-four-year-old Nancy an Aconcagua T-shirt signed by the members of Expedition Inspiration.

The next morning, Tuesday, January 31, after a silent prayer, the trek team assembled at Las Vacas Valley trailhead to begin its journey to base camp. Claudia Crosetti followed in Sue Anne's footsteps during the first leg of the hike. Later, Claudia wrote in her journal, "Her backpack has a small Earth flag sewn on it, the 'Spirit of the Trek Team' was sticking out of a side pocket, complete with wheat, her pack was tied with colorful straps and on her right foot a small, gold bell tinkled as we walked in the morning light."

Claudia continued: "The trek today was exactly what they told us it would be—lots of talus and scree. We had heavy winds, about fifty miles an hour, sometimes stronger. Nancy Johnson said she was afraid that we were going to lose Andrea Martin at one point. Andrea only weighs about a hundred pounds and the wind was blowing her off balance."

Patty, her limbs stiff from the effects of chemo-induced rheumatoid arthritis, had a hard time keeping her footing in the wind's assault. "Once, after losing my balance, I went forward, stepped on a loose rock and totally buckled under," she recalled. "I curled under and rolled and landed on my right shoulder and back. I twisted my left leg, which really hurt. I thought, 'Please God, I don't want to be hurt now.' But it was okay after about ten minutes. I was a little stiffer than usual the next morning. I was thankful that it wasn't worse."

In another journal entry, Claudia Crosetti wrote, "On the last leg of our trek today, Nancy Hudson couldn't hold back her enthusiasm any longer and took off ahead of Tuck and the rest of the team. He let her go, but had some words with her later. He was pretty nice to her about it. He said, 'Nancy, don't you like us anymore? Don't you want to be with the team?'"

Before the climb, Nancy had wanted to be moved to the summit team, but she had no climbing experience. Athletic and motivated, she was determined to climb at least to high camp at 19,000 feet, and was full of conflicting emotions about her own personal goal versus the team's goal. This conflict, added to the turmoil in her personal life, manifested itself in a nightmare in which her two sons had been kidnapped. On the second morning of the trek, she awoke crying and cried throughout the morning, while various team members tried to console her.

She later told Claudia Crosetti, "I think a lot of feelings I've been holding in about my cancer, my family, the divorce and the boys came out under the stress and emotion of the trek. Maybe altitude is part of it. I think your brain kind of goes cuckoo up in altitude. I think this has been good for me. I can be a little testy at times. I always want to go up one more step, go a little faster, and I have to learn patience, which I don't seem to have a lot of."

Andrea Martin said she was learning patience trying to negotiate the trail. "One step at a time never meant so much to me as it did on this trek. There is nothing you can do to prepare yourself for stepping on all these rocks. Every once in a while I got into a zone and I almost flitted from rock to rock and that lasted for maybe fifteen seconds, followed by about five minutes of klutziness. It's really a transferable lesson, because if you take this kind of awareness into your normal, day-to-day life, you realize that we all could slow down a little bit and possibly accomplish more."

Sara, the oldest of the survivors—as she liked to remind her teammates—had no problem trekking. The team could always count on her for a calm and positive outlook. Sara pronounced each river crossing "a piece of cake" and added, "Fortunately, the body is cooperating. The mind is another thing. I found I really had to get myself totally psyched up for this. It's been hard, because I don't have anyone home in Wisconsin with whom I can even discuss this except my husband, who is a saint. My friends can't figure the whole deal out. It's very hard to draw the line between it being an ego trip and a force for good. I think certain friends have had a problem with that. It's no ego trip for me. I'm delighted that the media is covering it, but there are more important things in my life than the media. I am so impressed with the women on our team—no nit picking or whining. I think our experience on Rainier was good. It really got the kinks out. I think we're a fabulous group of people!"

On February 1, the second day of the trek, the winds blew even harder. Nancy Johnson wrote in her journal: "The whole day was hard, physically and emotionally. It was the longest day, but also during the windy parts some people actually almost blew away. Ashley blew over—I held onto her—and Kathy Grant almost went over. Even Roger, who's over six feet tall, got blown back a step or two. I was watching how we were all struggling in the wind and it really brought up for me how we all have struggled with cancer and how other women are struggling. It was an emotional day and an analogy for me. It reminded me of the whole purpose of the climb—to inspire women—and also that a lot of women don't survive. We're here to be an inspiration to women who may have just been diagnosed, or have had surgery or are going through chemotherapy. Those women have their own windy days, the kind when you just feel like giving up. You feel terrible, you don't want to go on. But today we did go on. We took one step at a time and we made it to camp. For those women who are out there struggling with breast cancer, I hope that our efforts will encourage them to take that extra step, to hang in there and survive."

Nancy added, "Just before our second camp, when we saw Aconcagua for the first time on the trek, and saw all the weather up there, it also made me think of how the summit team must be struggling and made me anxious to hear from them."

After the trek team had settled in at Casa de Piedras, Tuck received a quick radio transmission from Peter, who was waiting out the storm at Camp 1 with the summit team. As we had done on Mount Rainier, the teams took turns exchanging cheers to send each other energy.

Then Peter said, "Tuck, we're carrying to Camp 2 tomorrow, no matter what the weather. This storm can't last."

Tuck replied, "Okay, we're sending good energy for warmth and no wind for the ascent."

Later that evening, the trek team had a sobering moment when two disoriented Slovenians wandered into camp, asking, "Are we in Chile?" Apparently they had summited, but then abandoned all their gear in the storm in order to descend the mountain quickly. They had been lost, without food or shelter, for several days. Mark Tucker, the Shepherd, gave them food, sleeping bags and a tent to use for the night.

The next day, February 2, during the trek team's approach to base camp, Patty collapsed about an hour out. "I got a horrible headache, I felt numb from the knees down and tingly all over," she later told me. "I think the spell was brought on by a bad hot flash."

Dr. Ron and Ned stayed with Patty while Tuck led the rest of the team to base camp. Dr. Ron made Patty lie down on the ground until the tingling sensation had passed. He said, "Just wait out the cycle. We're in no hurry." As soon as she started to rally, he made her drink water, eat some chocolate and put on warm clothes. Then they started walking again.

Meanwhile, the trek team arrived in base camp to the cheers of other climbers camped there. Claudia wrote in her journal, "I walked into base camp behind Eleanor. She turned and grinned at me as other expeditions cheered us. At camp, Nancy and I hugged—we had worked out together for fifteen months, and now, here we were! Jeannie Morris hugged each one of us and gave us notes from the summit team members. To the whole trek team, Claudia B–S wrote, 'I think of you all the time—you're pushing me up the mountain. Kick back and relax; it's awesome here. Celebrate your wellness."

Andrea Martin stated, "Six years ago, my doctor advised me to go home and put my affairs in order. Now, here I am at Aconcagua base camp. Incredible!"

Kim had a hard time tearing herself away from Patty and going on to camp with the team. "It was so hard to leave her," Kim said. "We'd been tenting or rooming together throughout this whole project and had become good friends. I knew she was in good hands, but I knew how badly she wanted to make it to base camp."

Patty, Ned and Dr. Ron finally cleared the ridge and came within sight of base camp. The team cheered them the rest of the way in. Patty began to cry as her teammates surrounded her with hugs and Kim handed her a mug of hot chocolate. Suddenly, Patty broke into a smile and looked directly at the PBS camera. She had a special message for her husband, who had feared she would never make it this far: "Hi honey, I'm in base camp!"

Patty later told me, "Before the climb, my sister gave me some great advice. She said, 'Take your heart and throw it up the mountain. Then follow it.' That's what I did. That's what got me up there."

Erika and Tuck were elated. Erika said, "Seeing everything come together like this makes me feel so good, because it has been so much work for everyone. Being with this group is very spiritual. Life means so much. I can't believe how well everyone has done."

Tuck added, "Getting to base camp takes off a lot of pressure. I think we're looking good. We're in position. What impresses me about this group is that they've already hurt big time in their lives, so they know how to just suck it up and gut it out. That's what climbing is all about—you've got to endure. The rewards aren't so tangible for some, but are overwhelming for others. I think we have a group that can really appreciate the pure essence of what we're doing."

With an odd number of team members, Sue Anne had volunteered to tent alone, much to her delight. At base camp, she painted "Massage Parlor" on her tent and announced that she was open for business: "for massage, games, creative arts, meditation and prayers for the summit team." She planted the prayer arrow and spirit stick outside the entrance to her tent, and was rarely without a customer.

Sue Anne told Claudia Crosetti, "Before the trip, I had a vision in which I felt a ram merge with me. It told me, 'I will help you go the distance.' I felt that something butted me up this mountain. Never once did I feel that I wouldn't make it. I never had the fear of failing that I had on Rainier. During those really windy days, it was amazing to me, because I have always tried to get out of the wind. The wind scrambles my energy, but there was no way to get away from it. So I sort of got into it and I let myself be whipped around and moved into it and I finished that day on some kind of a high. I practically leaped into camp. It was pure emotional power."

Ashley confided to Claudia that Tuck had called her before the trip to talk about looking at the climb as a team effort rather than her own personal goal and achievement. "Tuck said that whatever decisions were made about going higher than base camp were dependent on what was for the good of the team," said Ashley. "He said that we were there to support the summit team. Our conversation turned me around completely. I was relieved that I didn't have to prove anything to myself or to my community by trying to reach some personal goal. I could go and be supportive in whatever way I was needed."

Eleanor called on the support of friends who had passed away to give her strength on the expedition. "A friend I had known since high school, Carol, had survived a liver transplant for seven years, then got pneumonia and died in January, just before we left for Aconcagua. I kept her sitting on my right shoulder. I felt she was still connected to the earth, and her energy was all around me. And all the patients, all the friends of mine who have died of breast cancer, and another friend, Beverly, who was in the hospital during the climb—I asked them all to help make my feet light, make my pack light. It gave me joy to think of them and made it easier to climb the mountain. It also made me realize how fortunate I am to be healthy and not to be fussing about the difficulty but to revel in the experience and make the pain also part of the living, part of the experience."

For Roberta, the trek to base camp was "beyond any kind of wild dreams I've ever had," she said. "It's more spectacular, more beautiful, more intense, more rewarding, more stimulating, more exciting, more emotional, more *everything* than I had anticipated. Thank God for the rest-step and pressure breathing! When we got to base camp, I wasn't so completely exhausted as I was on Rainier. I was one of the first people to arrive in base camp, which was an extremely rewarding experience. All that working out really paid off for me."

Roberta added, "There were a few times when I could feel that I was running out of energy. I could feel my legs getting weak and my heart pounding, and I'd start having doubts and the image of that pale, skinny, wimpy kid who never got picked for the team would sneak back into my mind. At those moments I kept remembering all my friends and family and loved ones back home. I could feel their energy and their strength on my back, pushing me up through those moments. I could hear their words, 'You can do it, you can do it. Keep doing it.' Thanks to them and the guides' instruction and all this sisterhood that we're experiencing, I did it. I'm not the token wimp anymore!"

Nancy Johnson was reminded of a discussion among several of the trek team members before their departure for Argentina. "We often asked ourselves, 'Why did we survive breast cancer and other women didn't?' We realized we all feel similarly about wanting to give back. We feel passionate about the breast cancer issue. The fact that we bonded so quickly led us to believe that we were meant to meet each other and to do this climb to raise awareness. But I don't think any of us realized how big this was going to get and how much awareness we were going to raise."

It took climbing a mountain to find out.

The following morning, February 3, the trek team gathered in a circle, connected by the streams of prayer flags they had carried up the mountain and now held in their hands. In unison, they raised the flags above their heads. Each survivor took a turn reading names on the flags, four hundred names in all, a fraction of the total number of victims of the disease. The wind whipped up the team's energy and emotion, and carried into the ether the prayer inscribed on each flag: "*May the winds bring healing. May the winds bring serenity and remembrance. May we be free from illness.*"

Afterward, Dr. Ron remarked, "It's pretty sobering when you realize the magnitude of what we're tackling here. Even before we got on the mountain, we saw people coming through Puenta del Inca with frostbite, pneumonia and pulmonary edema. I knew this was going to be a physical challenge, but I guess what has really struck me in a good way is the emotional challenge of the trip. Being in the field of oncology, I have some idea of everybody's thoughts, but I didn't really anticipate such an emotional experience. With this team, there is something every day that really grabs you—and, to me, that can be more draining than the physical part. Roger and I were saying the other night that the guides chosen for this trip are very appropriate. Probably at no other time in their lives are you going to see these guides so emotionally brought to tears. There isn't a man on this trip who hasn't cried at any one of the events. It shows the power of what's going on. The prayer flag ceremony grabbed everybody."

At that point more grabbing news came over the radio: two members of the summit team were turning around and heading back down. Tuck and Ole were dispatched to Camp 1 to escort them safely to base camp.

On that morning, the summit team had awakened at Camp 1 to a clear, cold and nearly windless day—a perfect day to move to Camp 2. It wasn't so perfect for Mary and me. We had made the decision to return to base camp. Mary knew from her experience the day before that she could not climb any higher. I had developed congestion during the night and now my face was swollen. When Laura saw me, she said, "You look like a puffer fish." Peter took one look and said, "You're done."

Once the decision was made, it was easy to turn around. My purpose on the climb was to record the story and to provide support to the summit team. I knew if I tried to go higher and failed, one of the guides would have to bring me back down. I also knew that the loss of a guide could jeopardize the team's success and I was not willing to risk that possibility. There would be other summits for me, as there would be for Mary.

For the past three days, we had been pinned down by a blizzard at Camp 1. It had been a challenge to keep ourselves occupied inside our tents for fifteen hours at a stretch. Anticipation and anxiety filled our thoughts but went unexpressed as we waited out the storm. We'd go outside to pee—or, as Mary quipped, "You don't pee in this wind, you spray"—and then we'd rush back inside our tents. The wind increased the chill factor and made it too uncomfortable to stay outside for any length of time. A couple of team members had tried peeing in their tents in an extra water bottle or plastic bag, but found that the inevitable spillage did little to enhance their stature as agreeable tentmates.

We tried to sit outside in the mornings during the calmest part of the day. We'd huddle together behind a rock wall and eat breakfast—usually, bagels with peanut butter and jelly, and hot tea or coffee. When the cold eventually seeped through our four layers of clothing, we crawled back into our tents to read books, write in journals, play cards, snack and sleep.

At the time, I noted in my journal that I was steadily losing appetite and having trouble making myself eat—symptoms that should have rung some alarm bells, but didn't. Claudia B-S, on the other hand, effortlessly wolfed down second helpings. Mary seemed to be eating normally, but except for her cough, she had become unusually quiet.

Laura and Annette slept, read and wrote. "We were good tentmates," Annette noted. "In some ways, we are polar opposites. Laura tends to get diarrhea; I get constipated. She pees every forty-five minutes; I have the largest bladder in the world. We are both okay with being quiet, so it was no problem spending so much time together in the tent. Laura is organized and keeps all her stuff divided into little stuff sacks, while my stuff seems to spread out and take on a life of its own. I did manage to keep all of it on my side of the tent. It wasn't hard to tell which side of the tent was Laura's and which was mine."

Vicki and Nancy Knoble's tent was perched behind a huge boulder and therefore was more shielded from the wind. Vicki had developed a swollen gland in her throat, and Nancy's eyes were red and puffy from an allergic reaction to some substance. Thinking the culprit might be her down-filled sleeping bag, she traded it for Claudia B-S's synthetic-insulated bag and her symptoms gradually subsided. Despite their afflictions, both Vicki and Nancy maintained positive spirits.

We grew accustomed to the noise of the wind pounding and shaking the tents. When the wind quieted down, we'd jerk awake. Soon we'd hear a rumble building again in the distance, whipping off the peaks above us, rushing down into the valley, scouring the ground and nearly flattening our shelters.

When we awoke on Thursday, February 2, to light winds, we knew the carry to Camp 2 at 19,000 feet was a go. We loaded our packs with half our food and gear and started climbing, single file, behind Peter. As soon as we reached a snow-covered ridge at 17,500 feet, the wind whipped up again and began to knock us around. Maintaining a steady pace was difficult. We'd take a few steps forward, then brace ourselves as a gust hammered against our bodies and broke our tempo. Then we'd move on again until the next gust rammed into us. We were dressed in thermal underwear, insulating fleece sweaters and windproof Gore-Tex jackets and bib pants, plus insulated, windproof hats and gloves. Even so, the cold seeped in and took its toll.

Mary turned around with Kurt at 17,000 feet. None of us noticed until we reached a rest break around 18,000 feet. Somebody asked, "Where's Mary?"

"She decided to go back to camp," Peter said, and changed the subject by reminding us to drink lots of water and eat something in preparation for the next stretch. Peter never dwelled on negative thoughts. He told me later, "Whenever anyone faltered or had to turn around, it tore at my gut. I wanted to comfort and console them. Leaving the team and going in the other direction—man, I've been there. You've trained, you've made an emotional commitment, and then you have to split off. It's the worst feeling. But my job as leader is to keep the team going. At altitude, emotions run high. You can't afford to let spirits drop. You have to keep everyone else looking up, not thinking about going down."

We all said a quiet prayer for Mary, as well as one for ourselves. Annette and Vicki had fallen off pace on the way to this rest point and arrived as the remainder of the team was ready to push on to Camp 2. Guides John and Catie stayed with Annette and Vicki while they rested. I decided to remain a little longer there, too. My legs were cramping and I was coughing with congestion. At the time, I had no premonition that Mary and I would be turning around the next day and retreating to base camp.

John, Catie, Annette, Vicki and I reached Camp 2 about two hours later, gulping for oxygen. We had acclimatized to 16,200 feet. Tomorrow, when the team moved the rest of its gear to this new high camp at 19,000 feet, they'd have to acclimatize all over again. We dumped our gear and sat down on the ground for a quick snack. John laid out small portions of cheese, Pringles potato chips and Wheat Thins. I looked at the food and felt nausea rise in my stomach. My appetite was gone. I drank water and knew I would feel better as soon as we descended.

We had taken five-and-a-half hours to climb from 16,200 to 19,000 feet. On the way back down, John took us through a scree field and we slid on our feet most of the way, cutting the descent to ninety minutes. At one high point, we could see a long string of mules and people heading up the valley to base camp. John shouted to us, "It's the trek team!" They had narrowed our separation down to only a few thousand vertical feet. The sight of the team drawing nearer lifted our spirits as though we were being carried on the broad wings of condors.

The carry to Camp 2 had left all the summit team members burnt out and wind-battered. During the night, most of the team rested well and by Friday morning, most were anxious to move on. Having made the decision to descend to base camp, Mary and I made our good-byes and good-lucks brief. Then we watched our team members fall into place behind Peter and head off toward high camp.

Without Mary, only five breast cancer survivors remained on the summit team. Would the good weather hold another two days and allow the team to reach the summit? Or would the mountain conspire against Expedition Inspiration? All the team members could do now was act as though everything depended on them.

Mary and I retreated to our tent and worked on keeping our thoughts positive. Mary looked pale and drawn, but seemed to be in good spirits. "I think I've been struggling with oxygen deprivation," she said. "And this cough is wearing me out. Peter maintains a good pace that keeps the team together most of the time, but I had trouble going that fast. Yesterday, when I turned around with Kurt, I thought, 'I guess this is the time for me to bow out.' I probably could have kept going with Kurt, creeping at a snail's pace, and I might have gone up higher, but then I started thinking, 'Kurt could be used to help out up there.' A lot of thoughts went through my head. Kurt and I talked and I finally said, 'It's time for me to turn.' He started to walk back down to Camp 1. I said, 'Hold on, just a minute,' and I bowed my head over my trekking poles and let the tears come. After Kurt brought me back to our tent, he gave me a radio and made sure I had extra water. He explained that he was going to carry his load on up to Camp 2 and asked if I would be all right waiting here by myself. He was very caring and compassionate."

Mary added, "When you are with a team, you have to work

as a team. There isn't much room for individuality. Looking at it from my perspective, I don't know what other people would say or how they would decide, but I made the decision based on what I knew was right at that particular moment. You make a decision and live with it. That's it."

Mary and I tried to play cards to pass the time, but neither of us could keep our minds on the game. We kept starting over, redealing hands. I finally realized that it was a hopeless endeavor. "Maybe it's the altitude," I mumbled, shoving the deck of cards in my pack and retrieving a book instead. I felt as if I were in limbo, disconnected from both the summit and trek teams.

Finally, at noon, Mark Tucker and Ole Olson knocked on our tent door and greeted us with sandwiches and hugs. After we took a few bites—our appetites were still nominal—we put on our packs and followed the two men back to base camp. The trek team was waiting for us with open arms and lots of questions.

"Are you okay? Let me take your pack, eat some oranges, here's some water. How is Laura? What time did they start out today? Are they looking good? Is everyone healthy? Do you think they'll make it?"

As Mary said later, "It was like walking into the best support group anywhere!"

The trek team had spruced up base camp with thirteen new tents, hundreds of prayer flags streaming in the wind and banners hanging everywhere. The atmosphere was festive and charged with anticipation. Mary and I settled into an empty tent and considered Sue Anne's offer of a foot massage.

"That would be quite an olfactory challenge right now, don't you think?" I joked, pulling off a pair of socks I had worn for five days and throwing them outside the tent.

"I think I'll wait until after I bathe tomorrow," Mary said, tossing her socks in the same direction.

At dinner, Tuck announced that he had received a call from Peter, with the message that the summit team had made it intact to its 19,000-foot Camp 2 and was settling in for the night. "Peter is going to get up around three a.m. to monitor the weather," Tuck explained. "If it looks good, they'll try to get on the trail by five-thirty. We should get a call later in the morning, telling us whether or not they have left camp. It will take them a minimum of eight hours to get to the summit." Mountain gods willing, tomorrow could be summit day.

Most of the trek team members had come to Aconcagua with the goal of climbing higher than is possible in the continental U.S. (California's Mount Whitney is the highest point at 14,494 feet). Tomorrow, Saturday, on the same day that the summit team would try to reach the top of Aconcagua, the trekkers would attempt to reach their goal. Tuck informed the team that there would be two options: one group would get up at five a.m., before sunrise, and head for Camp 2; another group would leave later in the morning with the goal of reaching Camp 1. The first option involved climbing over five thousand vertical feet in one day—from 13,800-foot base camp to 19,000-foot high camp—an ambitious goal.

Tuck reminded everyone that if the summit team reached the top of Aconcagua tomorrow, they would then return to Camp 2 and spend another night there. The following morning, Sunday, Tuck would mobilize a group of guides and trekkers to intercept the descending summiters at 16,200-foot Camp 1, to help carry gear back to base camp.

When Tuck asked, "How many are interested in going to 19,000 feet tomorrow?" several team members raised their hands, including Nancy Hudson, Nancy Johnson, Dr. Kathleen Grant, Dr. Ron, Sue Anne, Claudia Crosetti and Saskia. Roger said that his heart wasn't in it; he wanted to save his energy for Sunday in the event a summit attempt was made and he could help carry gear down from Camp 1. Kim and the others agreed to wait and do the same.

Claudia Crosetti wrote in her journal that night, "Climbing over five thousand feet in one day? Would we then have the strength to climb to 16,200 the following day to help the summit team? Personally, I doubt it."

Mary and I encouraged the trek team members to climb as high as they could. "You'll enjoy the experience—and the view," we said.

I was surprised to see Saskia raise her hand for the hike to 19,000 feet. Several months before, she had switched from the summit team to the trek team because her busy work schedule was not allowing her the necessary time to adequately train for a summit climb. Now she had a bad cold and a rattling cough. I leaned over to her. "You won't get any better, going up higher. You could put yourself in danger." She smiled and said, "I'm fine. Really."

By morning, Saskia was not fine. Claudia Crosetti wrote in her journal, "Up at five-fifteen for our ascent. Great weather. We all felt good. Gear ready, outfitted in gaiters, fleece pants, Marmot windbreakers, headlamps, two gloves, light pack, layers, layers, layers. Then Tuck comes up to me as I was ready to get a hot drink and join the team and drops it on me: Saskia has pulmonary edema and has to be evacuated from the camp. Apparently, she came into the climb with a cold and congestion and never reported any symptoms to the guides or doctors, as they had asked us to do. According to Nancy Hudson, who's been tenting with Saskia at base camp, Saskia was up all night complaining of not being able to breathe and a headache as big as a mountain, but she didn't feel that she needed to see a doctor."

Early in the morning, Nancy Hudson had finally told Saskia,

"You're seeing a doctor. You've got to make a move." Nancy woke up Dr. Grant, who listened to Saskia's chest and heard gurgling in her lungs. The climb was over for Saskia.

Two guides, Ned and Larry, were mobilized to escort Saskia back to Puenta del Inca. There Ned would continue on to Mendoza with Saskia to find a doctor, while Larry returned to base camp. They took a radio in order to monitor the summit attempt, which, in all the confusion and concern over Saskia, had temporarily taken a back seat.

Nancy Hudson later told me, "I was up all night with Saskia and I was the one who wanted the most to go to 19,000 feet. I cried and cried. I was scared for Saskia and disappointed for myself."

Luckily, Saskia started feeling better as soon as she descended with the guides to Las Vacas Valley. We learned later that when she arrived in Mendoza, her condition had subsided to a cold again.

By the time Saskia and the guides had departed, it had grown too late to send a group of hikers up to 19,000 feet. However, Tuck announced, trek team members could still climb to Camp 1 at 16,200 feet. Tuck had received another call from Peter. The summit team had left Camp 2 at five-thirty that morning and had begun the ascent. Peter had called from a rest break at 20,500 feet, with both good and bad news.

The good news was that it was a beautiful summit day: clear, cold and no wind.

The bad news was that two more team members had turned around and were headed back to base camp with guides Kurt and Catie. According to climbing tradition, Peter did not give the names of the team members who were turning around, which left us in a state of suspended anxiety.

Tuck said, "I appreciate everyone being so flexible. You're a wonderful support team. We're going to work out the logistics here, so bear with us for the next hour 'til we get the program finalized. Let's keep doing what we can to keep ourselves strong and be team members who can help out, in case you're needed. So stay hydrated, fuel the furnace and relax." He grinned. "I know it's hard. I'm ready to jump out of my skin, but do what you can."

About an hour later, Ole led several trek team members up toward Camp 1, to intercept the descending climbers. Claudia Crosetti wrote in her journal, "At 15,100 feet, we met Kurt, Catie, Paul and Annette. It was emotional for all of us, but Paul and Annette looked strong. As we climbed back down to base camp, I could see the many beautiful prayer flags in the afternoon wind, and the whole team gathered on a ridge with Erika, who was holding the radio. It was four-ten in the afternoon. Peter had just called to tell us that they were a hundred and fifty feet from the summit."

Mountain of Hope

SASKIA'S EVACUATION FROM BASE CAMP, followed by Paul and Annette's return to base camp, had set the trek team's emotional pendulum swinging. We stayed close to each other, talking and occupying ourselves with simple tasks: helping to prepare food, rearranging gear, bathing, taking turns hauling water from the nearby glacial runoff. By four-thirty that afternoon, the entire team had gathered together on the ridge above base camp, expecting Erika's radio to burst forth at any moment with news from the summit.

The summit team had suffered through a long and grueling day. That morning, Peter had set his alarm for three-thirty. "As soon as I stuck my head out of the tent, I knew it was going to be good weather," he told me later. "Catie, Heather and Jeff were in the tent next to mine and John's. They had all the stoves with

195

them and I asked them to start melting snow for water. At that ungodly time of the morning, you get up, get dressed and hope you'll have time to have a hot drink.

"It was cold up there," he added, "at least zero degrees. We usually start for the summit later on Aconcagua than on Rainier because it's so cold. You don't want to set out before dark and then have to turn around just because you're cold.

"Bud came over to my tent about a half-hour after everyone was awake and told me that Paul wasn't going. I wasn't surprised. I had talked to him the night before and knew he was hurting." Paul had developed a sinus congestion that had worsened at altitude.

Bud told us how hard it was for him to leave Paul. "As Jimmy and I were getting up and getting dressed, I looked at Paul and he was lying there, flat, staring at the top of the tent. He kind of did one of those things where you move your eyes to look to talk to somebody, but you don't move your head. He said, 'I'm not going. I can't go.' It was obvious that no questions needed to be asked. Paul knew that he was done. It was deflating to me because Paul really wanted to go and we had talked a ton about it and we were doing everything together. It took a lot of my energy away at that moment. On the climb, when one of us would have a sinker, the other would pull him up, usually with a laugh or some humor and that had really worked for us. This time was different. I told Peter. Peter came over to Paul and said that Catie would stay with him."

Paul told me later, "I knew I could have started out with the team, but I didn't feel I'd be a contributor. I wanted to contribute. I wanted to help the team get to the summit. I realized I might have put somebody else in jeopardy from going to the top. If it had only been me, I could have taken another day, rested up, and gone on. But, it wasn't only me, it was the team."

Three rope teams left Camp 2 for the summit: Peter, Laura, Claudia B–S and Bud; John, Nancy Knoble, Vicki, Annette and Kurt; and Steve, Jeff, Heather and Jimmy.

"The one mistake I made was *really* a good one," Peter recalled, wryly. "I should have marked the route out of camp with wands the night before, but I forgot. When you leave Camp 2, you go downhill a little bit at first before you start going up again on the traverse. There's a water source that runs down there and forms large holes beneath the snow and among the *nieve penitentes*—snow pillars up to several feet high produced by a combination of wind, solar radiation and snowmelt. When new snow falls, as it had during the three days we were stuck at Camp 1, it covers the holes and spaces between the penitentes. I knew they were there; I just forgot about them. The ground looks smooth, and then you step out there and—*poof!*—you fall right in.

"Well, that's what happened. Within three minutes of leaving camp, I'm waist deep, sternum deep in places, punching through these holes in the snow. It was still dark, so the people behind me didn't see it happen and they all went in, too, one right after the other. You had to roll out of the hole and struggle to stand up; take another step and then down you went again. I shouted to John to take a lower route, and he did, but not low enough, so they fell in the holes, too. I'm thinking, my God, this is going to wipe out these people before we get five minutes out of camp. Heather, who was leading the third rope, actually went even lower than John and found a path that worked. I shouted to the other two rope teams that we had to roll downhill to this place that Heather had found. I mean, we were a mess of ropes and packs and bodies rolling down this hill. We spent almost a half hour of intense exertion at 19,000 feet before we even got started. Major mistake on my part."

Once on the trail, the team settled into a steady pace. "We'd been walking ninety minutes or so," said Peter, "and suddenly I heard Kurt shouting at me: 'I've got problems, Pete! Annette has to stop!' I unclipped from the rope and ran back. It was clear that Annette was finished. I decided to send Kurt back with her, so we unclipped them from their rope team and roped them together, turned them around and scrambled. It's always tough when you turn someone around. You want to keep things moving, but here we are again with the team splitting. And it's the first person to turn back on summit day. I really like Annette a lot—I picked her for the team—and it was tough to watch her go back."

Laura added, "It was sad because Annette thought she was letting me down along with so many others, which wasn't true. There would be other summits for her. But it made me sad to see her sobbing, gasping for air, and to know that after all her hard work, this climb was over for her."

Vicki said, "When Annette turned back, Nancy looked at me and said, 'There's only four of us. We've got to do this.' Reality set in, hard."

After Annette returned to base camp, she told me, "I wanted to go to the top, but I guess it wasn't my day. Everybody was feeling really strong when we first left camp this morning. After rolling in that snow, we started walking again and I suddenly felt as if no air would go into my lungs. Kurt looked at me and said, 'Tell me what you're feeling.' I said, 'For starters, my leg from the knee down feels like wood. My feet are icy. And I can't get any air.' That was it for me. Aconcagua's a big mountain; my hat's off to her. I hadn't eaten anything before we left camp, so by the time Kurt and I got back to the tents, I was on my knees on the tent floor ripping the wrapper off a granola bar and gobbling it down. Nothing has ever tasted so good. I had to take off my boots and socks and massage my feet for about an hour to get some warmth back into them."

It took the team three more hours to complete the traverse—"It was more like a long, steep, relentless incline," Laura said later—from Camp 2 to the point where the trail intersects with the Ruta Normal, an elevation gain of about fifteen hundred feet, all in new snow. By then, the sun had come up and Pete selected a spot on the shoulder of the mountain at which to take a break.

"I told everyone, face the sun and let it warm you up," he said. "We took a long break, almost forty minutes, to give everyone a chance to eat some food, drink lots of water and recuperate. Vicki and John took a little longer getting to the rest stop. I could see that Vicki was starting to fade, but at this point, everyone was frazzled. We radioed the team in base camp and when we heard the cheers from all our team members, our spirits were really boosted. Hearing them helped us an awful lot, helped move us along."

Knowing that the next two to three hours would be easier going, with less exposure to danger and less snow, Peter unroped the teams and set a slow, steady pace. "We used our ski poles and stayed together," he recounted. "Vicki fell off pace and at the next break, around 21,500 feet, she and John were clearly far enough out to where a decision was going to have to be made. John went out ahead of Vicki and hiked up to me. He and Vicki had already talked and made a decision. He had come up to ask us to wait for Vicki, because she wanted to say good-bye and to wish us luck. The scene was real emotional. She and Nancy had been tentmates, which made it hard on Nancy, too. And another survivor was splitting off. That left three survivors: Nancy Knoble, Claudia B-S and Laura."

"I felt sad to see Vicki turn," Laura said. "I was extremely proud of her. She dug deep to keep going, but her pace would never have gotten her to the top and back down safely."

For Nancy Knoble, that was the worst moment of the day. "Vicki and I had made a pact," she said. "We were determined to go to the summit together. John said, 'Nancy you go on with the others.' Vicki and I cried and then Vicki asked me to carry her prayer flags on up with me. It was almost more than I could bear."

Later Vicki told me, "I tried to talk John into going to the summit while I stayed at that high point, but he wouldn't hear of it. To decide to turn around at that point was really tough. But I loved standing that high in the Andes and being able to see and almost touch the summit. The decision was hard, but it was the right thing to do. Instead of telling me to buck up, John put his arms around me and held me while I cried. I felt so safe. I didn't feel stupid or ugly or any of that. I felt uplifted and I felt someone truly understood the pain of not making your goal."

From this point, the team had to make another traverse into a steep, rocky chute known as the infamous Canaleta. The Canaleta is a 1,300-foot-high, thirty-three-degree-angled chute of scree and loose rock. This season, the rocks were sporadically covered with fresh snow.

"The trail goes pretty much straight up, but we would have been more comfortable if we had been able to switchback up through the Canaleta," said Peter. "I tried to switchback a few times, but my feet plunged through the snow. On steep stuff, that's really draining work. We didn't need any more of that. So we roped up again, headed straight up in the snow and slowed way down. We used a lot of French technique—you turn sideways to the hill, put one foot above the other, roll your ankles and lock the downhill leg. Laura was slowing down here, having some problems." Peter kept reminding the team to "shake out your arms, make sure your shoulders are loose, take deep breaths, take one step at a time."

Nearly three hours later, the team emerged from the Canaleta. Everyone shed their packs and carried their water bottles inside their jackets the rest of the way. "The last part is an eight-hundred-foot struggle," said Peter. "There are places where you have to lever up. It's steep and unbroken with no opportunity for rhythm because the footing is so mixed. In some places, we'd take a few steps, then stop and do some pressure breathing before we could move on again. Instead of a nice summit ridge, it's an excruciating little crawl to the summit."

Jimmy, our photographer, described the climb to the summit as "really heinous. I was so oxygen-starved that I felt I was in a constant state of euphoria. A cloud would drift over and change the lighting and you'd think it was the first time I had used the camera. It was all I could do to concentrate on taking pictures."

Laura, Claudia B-S and Nancy Knoble concentrated on their goal. "I remember looking up at the summit or where the summit must be hidden behind rocks and boulders, thinking it would be a tough push," said Laura. "No rhythm. It would be important to keep the mind focused on the goal. I knew I had it in me and, of all climbs, on this one I knew I must stand on the top."

"There was a time when I had to dig deep and pull on my reserves," said Nancy Knoble. "I kept repeating my mantra— 'Confidence, Courage, Strength, Joy'—and the names of the women to whom I had dedicated the climb—'Cathie, Becky, Sharon, Francine.' I kept repeating that as I climbed. There never was a moment when I felt the toughness was getting overwhelming. I think I simply didn't want my mind to think about what my body was experiencing."

"There was no time when I thought I wouldn't make it," said Claudia B-S. "I didn't need to keep myself motivated. I had been motivated since Rainier. But the climb was very difficult.

During that last stretch above the Canaleta, we were taking pressure breaths two or three times per step and still getting tired. We came to a point with a great view of the South Face—10,000 feet, straight down. Pete called the trek team on the radio and when he heard Erika's voice he started to cry. So did the rest of us, but it was so great to hear the voices of our team. We could see the top from there. It looked close."

So close, yet still so far away. As the support team waited on the ridge above base camp in anticipation of Peter's next radio call, a burst of static shattered the air and sent us all jumping to our feet. I patted Roger's knee—he was trembling all over—and said, "Hang in there." He said, "I just want to hear her voice."

At four-thirty-five on Saturday, February 4, 1995, Peter's voice rang out: "We're five feet from the summit! I'm leaving the radio on the rest of the way." Erika held up the radio so that we could listen to the crunch of boots on rock as the team climbed to our long-awaited goal. Erika cried into the radio, "We are sending our breaths and our strength to you. Come on, you guys, two more steps. You can do it!"

Peter's voice rang out again, "We're on top!"

Base camp reverberated with cheers. We linked arms, crying and laughing with relief as the past two years' work ascended to a final, triumphant moment.

Peter's voice, ragged with emotion and exhaustion, rang out again. "We picked a big mountain. This is a huge hill of hope, but we did it. We're on top!"

"This is the moment everyone has been waiting for, for two years," Erika responded, her voice also quavering. "We're right there with you. We love you so much and we'd really like to hear from all of you, just a word, so we can hear your voices."

Laura came on the radio. "This is the toughest thing I've ever done since surviving cancer, I'll tell you that. It was rough."

Nancy Knoble: "This is truly amazing. We couldn't have done it without you. You're with us, absolutely, in our spirit, and we cannot wait to see you."

Claudia B-S: "I heard you pushing us up here. We wouldn't have made it if you hadn't been pushing. This is the toughest thing I've ever done."

Laura added, "We're standing up here in honor of all women, especially all the women who have suffered through breast cancer, as we have. And we're doing this with all our hearts and souls."

Erika handed the radio to Roger. "We're so proud of you," he said. "This means so much. You've carried every one of our dreams up to that mountain and made them all come true. We love you. You couldn't have done anything in your lives more important than what you have just accomplished."

Laura responded, "I'll tell you, we busted our butts to do it! We love you all so very, very much."

"We started walking eleven hours ago," said Peter. "We haven't eaten much food. We're about out of water. And we're looking at another four or five hours to get safely back to our high camp. I want everyone in base camp to realize that we couldn't have done this without your support."

We sent back a loud cheer, chanting the names of our summiters. Dr. Bud came on the radio and announced, "You guys have made us cry until we can't breathe. We have to stop."

It was time for Peter to resume his role as the General. "This is Expedition Inspiration Summit Team. We're shutting down and heading down."

We called out, "Be safe!" and reluctantly turned off the radio.

The entire team at base camp stood in one big circular embrace and rejoiced. Tuck, our Shepherd, grinned, his eyes brimming with tears. "Wow!" he said. "What am I going to do for kicks from now on?"

On the descent from the summit, Laura tripped and took a nosedive in the Canaleta. Peter rushed to her side, and was relieved to find her unhurt, but emotionally exhausted.

"I had an emotional meltdown," Laura said later. "All the effort—mental, emotional, physical—that had gone into this project, the underlying stress. All that evaporated on the summit."

Laura's resilience was still intact, however, and she quickly rallied. "I knew the climb wasn't a success unless we all got off the mountain safely," she said. "The rapid descent was good. It forced us to keep moving, to not think about fatigue or anything else, only moving safely down."

The summit team arrived back at Camp 2 at eight-thirty that night, after a three-and-a-half-hour descent. Fifteen hours had elapsed since starting out that morning. John and Vicki spotted the team on the traverse, and started boiling snow for hot drinks and dinner. As each summiter straggled into camp, John and Vicki helped them take off their gear and gave them a hot drink and food.

"To be there to help the team bonded me to them in an important way," said Vicki. "I needed to do that."

Laura headed for her tent immediately, before she thought to take off her pack. Stuck in the doorway, she laughed and shed the pack. Then she took a few short minutes to gobble down a dinner of rehydrated lasagna and a hot drink, and by nine o'clock, she was in her sleeping bag for the night. "I felt such relief as I drifted off," she recalled, "such pride that the project had gone so well. I remember thinking on the summit, 'It has been five years since I was diagnosed with breast cancer. If I can do what I've just done, I must be cured.'"

The following morning, the team members in base camp mobilized to meet the summit team. A cadre of guides hit the trail to high camp before dawn, to help the summit team carry down its gear. At eight-thirty, Nancy Johnson, Claudia Crosetti, Nancy Hudson, Ashley, Sue Anne, Dr. Ron, Dr. Grant and Roger took off with guide Jen to intercept the descending climbers at Camp 1 and split up the load even further. Eleanor, Roberta and Andrea Martin climbed to 15,500 feet and waited there to greet the returning team.

Those remaining in base camp busied themselves with various tasks in preparation for the party that night. Three new people had joined us in base camp: Mary Yeo's daughter, also named Mary, her fiancé, and Judith Powell, another friend of the team. They would join the celebration, then descend with us.

We had two reasons to celebrate: the success of Expedition Inspiration and Claudia Crosetti's forty-second birthday. One of the many life events this group had gained appreciation for was birthdays. As one survivor explained, "All of us have stared hard at the alternative."

Thanks to the mules' carrying capacity, champagne, beer and the ingredients for two giant strawberry cheesecakes filled the base camp larder. Catie whipped up the cakes while others gathered snow from the mountain to pack into the two large ice chests that held the party libations.

Kim and Patty used the rain fly from the demolished base camp tent to design a party dress for Claudia Crosetti. Kim sat at the door of Claudia's tent and painted a watercolor of base camp, "to remind her of the view from her tent." The team members signed the back of the painting.

At three-thirty that afternoon, a long string of climbers appeared on the ridge above base camp. We waved and cheered, as we had done on Mount Rainier. One by one, the returning climbers made their way across the rocks into camp. From hospital to hilltop, it had been a long journey to this moment of reunion. At last, sharing hugs, tears and laughter, the team stood together again on the mountain.

That night, base camp rocked. After dinner and congratulatory speeches, we sang "Happy Birthday" to Claudia, presented her with Kim's watercolor and forced her to model the tent dress.

"This is the best birthday I'll probably ever have," said Claudia, "but the worst dress. Who wants the first dance?"

Peter, our beloved General, cautioned everyone about drinking alcohol at altitude. "Half a Dixie cup of champagne can put you right on your butt up here," he said. "Pace yourselves. Remember, we've still got to walk out of here." Suddenly, he grinned. "We've got plenty of medical professionals up here, so I'd recommend two or three glasses each!"

"I'll drink to that!" someone shouted and the revelry began.

We set up a boom box. Annette asked me to slip in a Tina Turner tape and turn on the power when she gave the go-ahead from her tent. Ten minutes later, her arm snaked out of the tent and waved at me. I punched the "play" button and Tina's "What's Love Got To Do With It" filled the air.

Annette and Eleanor emerged from the tent clad in minidresses, fishnet stockings, spiked heels, sequined eyelashes and blue and green fright wigs. They gyrated to the music until the heels on their shoes disintegrated in the scree. We whooped and hollered and shouted for more. Eventually, everyone joined in the dance—including the Argentine ranger and other climbers in base camp. In more ways than one, Expedition Inspiration would leave a lasting impression on Aconcagua climbing history.

We celebrated our good fortune and success under a canopy of brilliant stars against a backdrop of mountain ridges backlit by a bright moon. The following day while we organized and packed our gear in preparation for the trek back to Puenta del Inca, the wind began to nip at the tents again. After two days of perfect weather, dark clouds rolled in during the afternoon, and by night, snow had begun to fall. On the morning of Tuesday, February 7, Expedition Inspiration said farewell to a base camp blanketed in snow.

Even Mount Aconcagua knew how to show off.

The trek from base camp back to civilization at Puenta del Inca took only two days instead of the three needed to hike in. Peter moved us along at a brisk clip. The first day was the most grueling. The team, now totaling forty-two, traveled twenty-five miles in twelve hours—and suffered its first mishap.

Sue Anne tripped over a loose rock and fell, face forward, onto the trail. The impact knocked out the bridge holding her four front teeth and embedded part of one tooth in her lower lip. Dr. Bud deftly removed the tooth and treated the wound. Throughout the ordeal, Sue Anne remained unflappable, still high on the success of the team and enjoying every minute of the expedition. One of the gauchos volunteered to put her on his horse and lead her the rest of the way to camp. He grinned at Sue Anne to prove his sincerity and empathy: he was toothless, too.

In many ways, Sue Anne had been the keeper of the team's spirit, carrying the spirit stick and prayer arrow to base camp, gathering names for the Earth flag, nurturing other team members, always calling attention to the metaphysical side of the experience.

She had wanted to leave the prayer arrow at base camp in commemoration of the climb, but her plan had been thwarted.

"The guides swept base camp after we all left," she told me later. "At our first break on the trek out, one of them brought me the prayer arrow and said, 'You weren't supposed to leave any trash at base camp.' Instead of objecting to that statement and saying, 'This isn't trash, this is a *prayer arrow*, it's a very spiritual thing, it's important,' I started thinking about how else I could do what I wanted to do. Then, a miracle occurred.

"I took the arrow to our Argentinean guide, Ana, and explained what had happened. She took it to the gaucho who had led me out of Las Vacas Valley on his horse after I had lost my teeth. They spoke in Spanish, so I don't know what Ana said, but I could tell from the look on the gaucho's face that he understood immediately.

"He went into his tent and emerged with a condor feather, which he attached to the prayer arrow. He smiled at me, mounted his horse and rode off."

The gaucho galloped out of sight and rode deep into the canyon, far from trails and camps, far from human trappings. He rode with a heart full of purpose. When the prayer arrow left his hand, it sailed to a place of joy, a place where the sky is indistinguishable from the earth, where effort becomes effortless and where the hopes and dreams of the women of Expedition Inspiration live on forever.

Afterword

"We all loved each other—that made all the difference."
—Andrea Martin

Growth, Affirmation and Change

Claudia Crosetti closed her Aconcagua journal with this observation: "On the mountain, our normal worlds fell away. We were forced to communicate and work together based on nothing more than a mutual goal to get higher and to help each other survive. That which makes us who we are in our respective homes dissipated on the mountain. Finding ways to help one another as a team was not always easy, but was our goal. When we go back to our worlds, to our identities, to our loved ones, perhaps we'll go back with new insight."

Focusing on the expedition for over a year had consumed most of the team members' free time and energy. Families and friends had either rallied in support or taken a back seat until after the climb. Even with the insight gained from the expedition, re-entry into a "normal" life was a challenge for many team members. Many of them eased back into a semblance of normality while regularly presenting slide shows to various schools, support groups, businesses and cancer organizations.

The media coverage of Expedition Inspiration continued for several months. The PBS documentary premiered in the summer of 1995, and the entire team was honored at the White House, Congress and Supreme Court. Hillary Clinton introduced the team during her announcement of a new mammogram program. Members of Congress held a reception in the team's honor. And Justice Sandra Day O'Connor, herself a breast cancer survivor, gave the team members a personally guided tour of her chambers and the Court. In return, Nancy Knoble gave Justice O'Connor her Aconcagua team jacket.

Two weeks later, Paul Delorey flew the entire team to JanSport headquarters in Appleton, Wisconsin, for a weekend reunion. The town of Appleton opened its arms to the team, furnishing lodging and meals. Sara and Fritz threw a party at their house on Lake Winnebago. Paul and his wife, Sandi, took us whitewater rafting on the Wolf River and then back to their cabin for a cookout. Paul also introduced the team to the employees of JanSport, and singled out Sue Anne for a special honor called the Foster Award.

"Every year, from now on, the employees of JanSport will cast their votes for a woman who has shown the most courage and perseverance under the most trying circumstances," said Paul. "Our first honoree is Sue Anne Foster, after whom the award is named." Paul told the story of how Sue Anne lost her teeth. Sue Anne slipped off her temporary bridge and smiled, unabashed, at the audience.

"After losing my breast to cancer, my hair to chemo and my teeth to the mountain, it's very clear to me that who I am is not my body," she said. "Who I am is a daily mystery to solve—and I like the assignment!"

For Andrea Martin and Laura Evans, the project had become a full-time job. Having raised over one million dollars through

Expedition Inspiration, Laura and Andrea agreed to part ways to allow each to pursue the promotion of breast cancer awareness and fundraising according to her own vision. Laura's fund, called the "Expedition Inspiration Fund for Breast Cancer Research," is headquartered in Ketchum, Idaho. Andrea Martin and the Breast Cancer Fund remain in San Francisco. Both organizations have developed a full program of participatory hikes and climbs in various places around the country.

For most of the team members, Expedition Inspiration became more than a metaphor for their breast cancer experience. The expedition had also established a foundation from which their lives would go forward, and forged a bond that remains unbroken to this day.

"We all seem to use the climb as a catalyst for change in other parts of our lives," says Kim O'Meara Anderson, who filed for divorce from Art two years after returning from Aconcagua.

"When I came back from the expedition, it was as though I was in shock," Kim recounts. "I couldn't get back into my routine at work. Many of the other team members I talked to felt the same way. I had missed my family, but when I got home, I found myself needing my own space. The climb helped me prioritize and determine what is really important in my life. Art and I never got back into the comfortableness that we'd had earlier on. I knew that when I went on the expedition, I was taking a risk with my marriage, but it's like living your life after cancer—you can't not do things out of fear. We were at a point in our relationship where we were either going to separate or drive each other crazy. I didn't want my son to grow up in this sort of atmosphere.

"The climb was a healing journey," Kim adds. "I'm a very different person now because of the cancer and because of the Aconcagua experience. I think I'm a better person."

Most of the team members share the feeling that their lives have improved in many ways, most importantly in terms of focus. Laura states, "When I was going through my treatment, I summoned up every ounce of energy I had and focused on getting well. That was my singular focus. I got close enough to death to realize that it's a relief, a release. I don't have any fear of death now. I understand that it's part of the process of life and I know now when it comes it will be okay. Having such a close brush with death makes you realize that this is all you have, this moment. You've got to make the most of it."

Andrea Martin notes that climbing Aconcagua has added another layer of strength to her persona. "We all loved each other, you know. That made all the difference."

Andrea continues, "I think we can win the battle against breast cancer with more funding and focus. We've been battling cancer for twenty-five years and not winning the war. What the Breast Cancer Fund stands for is getting people to look at breast cancer differently, to ask new questions, to look at different treatments, different tests. One of the biggest messages is to empower women. Today, as much as we've got the light shining on this subject, it could go out at any time. We've got to keep the pressure on and get to the point where we take responsibility for our own health into the next century."

Nancy Johnson also feels that the climb empowered her. "I loved how the challenge of the climb made me live in the moment," she says. "It was very much like cancer in that way. The whole time I was going through my cancer experience, I lived very much in the moment. It wasn't such a happy, great moment, but it really put me into a wonderful, spiritual place. It was all about survival—both cancer and being on the mountain. Rest-stepping, pressure breathing, drinking water, eating enough. Constantly wondering, am I too hot? Too cold?

How's my energy level? Am I doing everything I can do to help myself stay well and survive? I loved how that felt. I felt thankful, alive and challenged. It's hard to constantly maintain this feeling in your everyday life, but it's easier now to bring myself back to that place."

Nancy wrote a grant proposal to extend the services of the Mendocino Cancer Research Center by establishing a sister center in Ukiah, California. If the grant is approved, she will serve as director of the center. In the meantime, in addition to her regular job as an energy consultant, she continues to volunteer her time for WECAN, the Women's Cancer Advocacy Network. WECAN is a group of forty women, all cancer survivors from four neighboring counties, who serve as advocates for women who have recently been diagnosed with cancer. "We don't give advice or tell them what to do," says Nancy. "We help them become better informed and we are there for them, twenty-four hours a day. We go with them to doctor appointments, hold their hand during treatment, listen, hold them when they cry. We've been there, shared the same cancer experiences. Hopefully, our presence eases their journey."

What Claudia Crosetti enjoyed most about the climb was the absence of focus on materialism. "You don't have your house, your car, your job," she notes. "All you have to rely on is yourself and how you act with people and with the team. That's all that mattered up there. You got to peel away those outside layers and concentrate on your essence.

"The other benefit is that I feel I have reclaimed my body. I regained a trust in my body that I had lost when I was diagnosed. It took me about a year to recover from my treatment and surgery. I never knew if my body, my immune system, would come back completely. When I got to 16,200 feet on Aconcagua and I still felt strong, I said to myself, 'I think you're okay now.'

I have more confidence in myself. I've been doing more public speaking, I've changed jobs, I've started writing again. There are a lot of things you're capable of doing if you put yourself out there beyond what you think you can do."

For Nancy Hudson, the expedition had been more of an emotional challenge than a physical one. "Overall, it was a growing experience," she says. "It doesn't really matter that I didn't get to try to climb to high camp. What's more important is that I feel I've grown a lot and there's been a transformation in my personality. I learned the hard way that the journey is the more important experience, not the summit. I feel more secure." In the spring of 1997, Nancy finalized her divorce and finally had her breasts reconstructed—by Dr. Bud, of course. At a team reunion at Roberta's house, everyone was eager to see the results. One team member exclaimed, "Nancy, you're sixteen again!"

Ashley Sumner-Cox, the youngest team member, returned to Missoula to finish college. "Before the expedition, I had expectations of where I was going to be on the mountain and how I was going to acquire all this spiritual knowledge and be a different person," she says. "Being part of the team helped me find some peace and self-confidence. After I got back, I walked a little taller. But the most important thing that happened to me is that I realized that this is what I want to do in my life. I don't know if I could have made it to the summit of Aconcagua, but I was very fit and strong. I know I want to live in the mountains. I want to climb." Ashley finished college in the spring of 1997 and went to work as a mountaineering guide on Oregon's Mount Hood.

Roberta Fama broke up with Kipp after Aconcagua. "Even though Kipp is a wonderful man and I cherish the time we spent together, I felt that in the long run, we would not end up together," she says. "Since Kipp was uncomfortable with my feelings, we ended our romance." For a year after the climb, Roberta continued to serve on the board of the Breast Cancer Fund. "Then I decided that I didn't want the role of a professional breast cancer survivor anymore. I wanted to concentrate on moving forward into other parts of my life, so I resigned.

"For me, the best part of the whole project has been getting to know the other women on the team and spending time with them," Roberta adds. "Every single one of them has such a gift, something wonderful to offer. And the sense of accomplishment was so good for me. I had so many doubts and so much anxiety. The fact that I did better than I ever thought I could was great."

One of Roberta's last entries in her Aconcagua journal read: "I was told that she was an ugly mountain, I was told she was just a walkup; both were far from the truth. My breath was taken away each time we were blessed by the sight of her. Strong, powerful, kind and accepting, this (summit) day Aconcagua was a woman's mountain. We began as two ... six to the summit and eleven on the trek. Knowing in our hearts the greater goal and purpose for us to be here—to scream out to all women that together you can accomplish great things in spite of life's tragedies. I have a connection with these women no one can comprehend. They have become part of my soul, my life, my purpose."

Vicki Boriack also returned from the climb with a new sense of purpose. She finally resolved her relationship with Larry. "We both knew it was over," she said. "It was just hard to let go." She also wrestled with her Aconcagua experience for many months before coming to terms with not having made it to the summit. "It's really hard when you feel you haven't reached your goal. Sometimes I feel I haven't succeeded at that many things in my life. I try to bring myself down to a more realistic level. Maybe I've done the best job I can do, being a mom. Maybe I did the best I could at getting through the trauma of breast cancer. But when it comes to athletics, I never was the best at anything. And being average was sort of accepted in my family. I've fought that averageness my whole life. I didn't want to be average.

"Looking back, I realize how much I got out of the climb. I learned so much. I feel the climb was part of my wellness dosage: 'take this pill, climb, and you'll be well.' It was so wonderful to be climbing for the spirit of women, and with the spirit of women, instead of merely climbing. Now young women look at me and say, 'You're healthy, you're young. If you can get it, so can I.' If this brings awareness to them to do self-breast exams and to be conscious about breast health, maybe even one of those women will find a lump early and will still be able to live a long life."

Vicki is now following a new path that allows her to help more women deal with health issues and receive better health care. After the expedition, the company she worked for was acquired by another company and Vicki's job was eliminated in the ensuing downsizing. Vicki spent several months looking for another job and was eventually selected to be director of the Women's Health Alliance in Santa Clara County, an organization that seeks to help underserved women gain access to health care. "I am no longer in a job that is an interim position," says Vicki. "The job I have now is more in line with what I care about."

Annette Porter also struggled to come to terms with her performance on the climb. "I've never not reached a goal I've set out to reach," she acknowledges. "It took me awhile to figure out that this experience had become an AFGO—Another Fucking Growth Opportunity. It was easy to say, before the climb, that I believed in the journey, not the destination. It was easy to say that I believed I'd get as far as the mountain would let me. I said those things. Philosophically, I believed them. And then, when I turned back on the mountain, I got to live them. The same thing happened during my cancer experience, with my spirituality. It put my beliefs to the test. When you can finally say, 'Yes, I truly believe this,' you are given a wonderful sense of strength.

"The other thing I realized is how lucky I was. I got great medical care. I got to pick my doctors. I got to pick treatments. I got to ask questions. So often I think how lucky I was not to have a child who I was supporting and not to have to worry about day care while going to chemo. I wasn't this poor woman who all of a sudden woke up with a mastectomy and had children to care for, a job to hold down and inadequate medical coverage. In the spectrum of things, my situation was easy. I am grateful. What makes me angry is all the arguments about rationing health care. In my mind, it's rationed now. It's rationed economically. People who can afford it have access to it and the people who can't afford it, don't. After I left the company I was with I had medical coverage for eighteen months and then no one would insure me. Health care mixed up with profitability is crazy."

Nancy Knoble's best moment on the climb was rejoining the team at base camp. "Reaching the summit was wonderful, but being together on the mountain with the whole team was what I had looked forward to for a very long time," she says. "I really believe that a small group of committed people doing what they believe in can change the world. Yes, we were ordinary people doing the extraordinary, but you don't necessarily know that while you're doing it. It has to do with following your heart and following a passion and being committed. For me, the climb transported me from a frenetic, sixty-hour work week to an almost ascetic simplicity. I felt an essential connection with the mountain, with the world and with life. I gained a new perspective. I decided to quit my job to have more flexibility in my life, and to have more time to help others."

Nancy Knoble quit her twenty-year career position a year after returning from Aconcagua. She formed her own human resources and consulting practice, concentrating on team building and leadership training for small-to-medium-sized companies. She calls her business, BLITS—Because Life Is Too Short. As Nancy explains, "This was something I had been saying for a long time but hadn't been living."

For Sara Hildebrand, the trek was "very peaceful." She comments, "If you don't ask your body to do something, how are you going to know what your body is capable of doing? I was pleased that I had no trouble. I slept well every night, felt great every day."

Sara has not missed a single team reunion, but regards Aconcagua as a "closed chapter." She adds, "I don't think anything will ever duplicate this expedition. I am amazed how this team continues to grow and benefit from being empowered by their breast cancer and climbing experiences."

Sara herself has been empowered. She continues to work on developing a breast clinic for her community and was appointed by the wife of the governor of Wisconsin to the Women's Health Foundation, "the first of its kind in any state," she says. She also has been appointed to the Women's Leadership Board at Harvard's Kennedy School of Government. In addition, she pursues a busy schedule of speech making on behalf of breast cancer awareness and research, which has included giving a speech in Washington, D.C., to a Small Business Administration gathering at which President Clinton also spoke.

"My head was really swollen after that experience," grins Sara. "Three days later, I had to give a speech at the Yonkers Mall in Manitowoc, Wisconsin. It was pouring rain. We ran an hour late. What do people do in Wisconsin when it rains? They go to the mall. There I was in the middle of the mall, talking, showing my slides of Aconcagua, with people milling all around. The Humane Society shows up with cats and dogs to give away, so there was all this barking and meowing. I laughed so hard. I thought, 'There goes the swollen head.' Back down to earth. Sometimes, I feel we dreamed it all."

Both Sara and Laura were honored with a Jonquil Award from Duke University after the climb. According to Audrey Chase, who spearheads the award program for Duke's Comprehensive Cancer Center, "The Jonquil Award is a symbol that there's always hope, there's always life. It is given to women who have made an impression in breast cancer research of some kind."

Laura was honored as the founder of Expedition Inspiration. Sara was honored for achievements in her local community. Sara explains, "I've been able to change the way mammograms are done in our area. Instead of going into the office and writing your name and address on an envelope so they can stick the results in it and mail your diagnosis in a week, you hear right then, before you leave the office. And if there is a question, you see the surgeon right then."

After the climb, Claudia Berryman-Shafer realized that she had come full circle in a year's time. "I went from being in good shape, race condition, through diagnosis and treatment for breast cancer and back to being in good shape, summit condition. For me, the year was really a celebration of wellness," she says.

Claudia B-S also resumed teaching the alternative classroom of underprivileged problem kids, simply because, she says, "I missed them."

She adds, "I have let the experience of breast cancer go. Answering questions or helping others doesn't involve reliving the experience, which I believe is not healthy. Once you can let go then you no longer fear or think about recurrent disease. Obviously, you still have to go to your checkups and remain vigilant regarding your health, but all women need to do that."

Despite everyone's best efforts to be positive and vigilant, the disease still persists and tragedy occurs. Claudia B-S lost four people to breast cancer within the two years following the climb, including a cousin and Connie, the friend who had given her a book of meditations to carry on the mountain. Connie's cancer was a recurrence, and she still had no insurance to cover proper treatment. Claudia took Connie to doctor appointments and was with her near the end. "By the time she died, it was a relief," says Claudia. "I worked my way through college on the night shift in a nursing home, and I had forgotten how I enjoy being with sick people. You get more in touch with what is important in life. And, Connie is a reminder that not all who have had breast cancer get to climb mountains."

After the climb, Eleanor Davis told me, "The threat of a recurrence is on everyone's mind. I've been 'out' over sixteen years now, and certainly I remember within the first ten years that the fear of a recurrence was always pretty close to the surface of my thoughts. Within a group of seventeen women, how long are they all going to survive? For all the survivors to show up in Argentina with no family problems, no deaths in families, no injuries and everyone in good health was a miracle."

Shortly following the team reunion in Wisconsin in May, 1995, Eleanor sent a note to the other team members. "Today is Memorial Day and I went for a walk in Valley Forge Park. The tall grass changed colors as the sunlight moved softly across the fields. As I walked I could see your faces silhouetted so clearly against the blue sky, the wind blowing through your hair, Mona Lisa smiles hiding future uncertainties. For some, the uncertainties will disappear quickly; for others they may remain a lifetime. I found myself weeping at the thought that I might not see all of you again. I miss you already. I wanted you to know how much each of you means to me and how much you have enriched my life. Your faces, the tears and the laughter, will always occupy a special place in my mind and in my heart."

Was this bittersweet sentiment a portent of the tragedies that were to follow? After two years of blissful and illness-free involvement in Expedition Inspiration, reality intervened. Two days before Christmas 1995, Eleanor's oldest son, Chris, was killed in a car accident on his way home from work. The following December, Annette's father succumbed to a sudden heart attack and her mother had to be hospitalized for Alzheimer's Disease. In May 1997, Nancy Knoble was diagnosed with a recurrence.

Eleanor had fought hard to survive breast cancer to be able to raise her children. The irony was nearly unbearable. And although the pain felt by all the team members was nowhere near the intensity that Eleanor, her husband, Hal, and their family felt, the death of thirty-two-year-old Chris devastated the team. Before Chris's death, Eleanor had told me, "Life isn't over until it's over. We have to be constantly reminded of that, don't we? I say this to everyone: 'I can't wait to see what happens next year.' They ask, 'Why? Are you going on another climb?' I say, 'No, it doesn't have anything to do with that. It has to do with experiencing the future.'" Eleanor, a bereavement counselor, sought the same help for herself and began the long climb out of despair, one step at a time.

When Annette's father died, she was living outside London with her fiancé, Sami, a man she had met while exploring a new career opportunity in photography. "I had to spend a month at my parents' home, making funeral arrangements and planning care for my mother," Annette explains. "The whole process plunged me into a deep depression. Sami was great, so supportive. Confronting all those old family issues that I thought I'd resolved during my cancer was so strange. Now, here I was, face to face with them again. It became Another Fucking Growth Opportunity. It was so hard to leave my mother by herself. My father had been the person who interpreted her universe for her. But during one visit with my mother, it suddenly became so clear to me where I got the will to survive. I realized she's a survivor, too." Annette needed several months to work through her depression. She finally began to focus on working out for a climb of Mount Kilimanjaro in the fall of 1997, a trip I organized with Peter Whittaker and Summits Adventure Travel. Annette says, "Physical exertion enabled me to start moving again, to make some positive changes, to move toward something positive."

Nancy Knoble was moving toward another positive project—leading a new group of breast cancer survivors up Alaska's Mount McKinley for the Breast Cancer Fund's "Climb Against the Odds" in June 1998—when she was diagnosed with a recurrence in May 1997. Only three-and-a-half years had passed since her original diagnosis. Because the tumor was small and estrogen positive, her doctors did not recommend chemo. But the presence of more signs of DCIS caused Nancy to elect to have a bilateral mastectomy. "My doctor had been very vigilant. She had me coming in every three or four months for checkups," says Nancy. "The tumor was actually smaller and younger than the original one. I felt that this was the second gentle knock on the door. I realized that I'd had seven breast operations in less than four years, including biopsies, implants and the lumpectomy. I'd spent months recuperating from these surgeries. I began to feel as if my breasts were ruling my life, and that's not who I am. I wasn't sorry to see them go. My goal now is *no more surgeries*!

"My body has produced cancer twice," Nancy continues. "That reinforces the value of knowing what's important to me, and doing those things that are meaningful." Nancy recovered quickly from the mastectomy. "My recuperation was far ahead of schedule. I know this is because I'm fit and strong, both physically and mentally. For me, McKinley is full speed ahead."

At the last team reunion in the spring of 1997, Sue Anne appeared to be lighter, brighter and happier—and also moving full speed ahead. "My experience with the team gave me a tribal connection and helped me out of the depression I'd been suffering for several years," she told me. "The energy and positive spirit of the group resonated within and activated a part of me that knew what was wrong but hadn't been able to generate change alone."

Sue Anne had become involved in building labyrinths and using them for therapeutic purposes. She and her husband, Gary, had built a labyrinth together in their backyard. "It's one of the places in our lives where we are in agreement," Sue Anne told me. "It's a beginning."

Sue Anne describes how the labyrinth works. "The labyrinth is a multi-dimensional mandala that draws our attention as we learn how to recreate sacred space. The winding, archetypal path combines the circle and the spiral, symbols of wholeness, unity and transformation. There is only one path to the center and once the choice is made to enter, the path becomes a metaphor and mirror for the journey through life and the therapeutic healing process. Deepak Chopra says, 'The labyrinth experience invites us to explore the mind/body connection as we strengthen the vision of a healthy planet supporting life among diverse communities.'" Sue Anne had clearly found her path.

Mary Yeo, who had initially kept her breast cancer experience to herself before joining Expedition Inspiration, also found a new path. She turned into a traveling, one-woman testimony to the power of positive thinking and perseverance in overcoming a life-threatening disease. Mary has been interviewed regularly by a local TV news station. She has organized and spoken at several fundraising events and often travels out of Maine to present her slide show and lecture on Expedition Inspiration. She also has continued her active lifestyle of skiing, hiking, bicycling and traveling.

"From the climb, I gained a better understanding of other women who have had breast cancer," Mary explains. "I've learned that there is a definite will to survive and these women prove it. Patty Duke has been a real inspiration to me. She's out there doing it, and she's hurting but she's not complaining. She's just doing it. The will to do something for a cause that helps others is really admirable."

"I feel that the message from Expedition Inspiration goes to everybody in a lot of different ways," says Patty Duke. "I believe that there is something above us, a greater power, that helps mold and congeal and make things happen. We may not like the things that happen, but sometimes they lead us to discover what we need to know, something that has to be uncovered before it gets worse. There is breast cancer. There are other cancers. There are tragedies so terribly devastating you feel you can't move on. The message we have to offer is that you can move on and get past the tragedy and do something meaningful—for yourself, and for others."

The success of Expedition Inspiration does not diminish the fact that, for many women, "the mountain" is sometimes too high, the goal too distant, the struggle too demanding. For many, the journey's end seems premature. For me, Expedition Inspiration has become an axis star that shines continuously in my heart, giving my life direction and purpose. I believe that our triumph on the mountain offers many lessons, most importantly this: the struggle is worth every step.

Acknowledgments

This book was a labor of love. I offer my sincere appreciation to all who contributed to the fruition of this project, including: Faith Conlon, my editor and publisher at Seal Press, for her honesty, encouragement and patience; to Deborah Kaufmann, for her empathy and astute copy-editing; to Holly Morris, the book's first editor, for her unfailing support; to Jeannie Morris, my understanding colleague, for her generous friendship; and to Joan Alvarez, editor-in-chief of *Outdoor Retailer*, for her feedback on the manuscript and sponsorship of the expedition.

I'm grateful to all my friends and business associates in the outdoor industry who generously donated product or funds to Expedition Inspiration. A special note of gratitude goes to Paul Delorey, president of JanSport, for funding the entire expedition and infusing the project with a greater sense of compassion and dedication.

To Pete Whittaker, Laura Evans and Andrea Martin, I give my sincere thanks for making me a member of Expedition Inspiration, and for adding an enriching perspective to my life. A special nod goes to Pete for his encouragement and help in the project. I look forward to more adventures, Pete! Laura and Andrea, may wellness and success accompany you in all your pursuits.

Lou Whittaker and Skip Yowell first took me up the mountain and got me hooked on climbing—thanks, guys! Ingrid

Widman and Erika Whittaker showed me class on the mountain. Catie Casson and Heather MacDonald demonstrated woman-strength. Mark "Tuck" Tucker showed all of us more than a little tenderness. To John Hanron, Kurt Wedburg, Jeff Martin, Sue Luther, Larry Luther, Jen Wedburg, Ole Olson and Ned Randolf, I thank you for your guidance and compassion. May all your climbs be roundtrips!

A special thanks goes to Barb Harris, editor-in-chief, and Peg Moline, editor, at *Shape* magazine for being up front in media support of the project.

Expressing the gratitude, pride and love I feel for each of the women of Expedition Inspiration is difficult because mere words are finite and my feelings are boundless. I thank all of them for sharing their homes, hearts and thoughts before, during and after the project, so that other women may benefit from their experiences.

To Nancy Hudson, Roberta Fama and Sara Hildebrand, thank you for so graciously hosting team reunions. To Dr. Bud Alpert, Dr. Ron Dorn and Dr. Kathleen Grant, thanks for your endless generosity.

Claudia Crosetti, thanks for being my eyes and ears on the trek team. May your writing career flourish!

Thanks to Claudia Berryman-Shafer and Mary Yeo, for being the best tentmates! Thanks to all the team members for sharing photos for the book.

To Eleanor Davis and Annette Porter, I am grateful for the "revival and rejuvenation" trips we took together and look forward to more.

Evan Anderson, you will always occupy a special place in my heart.

I will always remember the kindness and dedication of Jo Spencer and Janice Fish, who organized a fundraising hike of

Mount Inspiration in their home state of Kentucky, then journeyed to California to meet the team.

I am blessed with loving family and friends. My thanks to all of them. A special thanks to Sally Jeans for turning the awesome task of transcribing the interview tapes into a superb accomplishment; Arlene, Sharon and Pam for providing early feedback and unflagging support; Lacey, for pitching in during deadlines and giving me the music that makes me type; Dan, for computer rescue!

To Francey, my dearest friend and life partner, thank you for your patience and understanding and for encouraging me to pursue my dreams. You make everything worthwhile.

I send loving thoughts to my grandmother, mother, father-in-law and friend, Susan, who lost their battles with cancer, but went to the mountain with me in spirit.

A portion of the profits from the sale of this book is being donated to breast cancer research. Thank you for buying this book.

Sponsors

Adventure-16
Adventure Medical Kits
Basic Designs/Stearns
BTU Stoker, Inc.
Cascade Designs
Chaco
Champion Nutrition
Crazy Pad Covers
Duofold
DuPont Cordura
Early Winters
EFI
Eiler Communications
Elgin Syferd
GMR Marketing
JanSport
Leki-Sport USA
L.L. Bean
Malden Mills
Marmot Mountain, Ltd.
Mary Kay Cosmetics
MontBell America
Mountain Safety Research

Moving Comfort
Nalge
Northwest Airlines
Ocean Designs
Outdoor Research, Inc.
Outdoor Retailer
Petzl/PMI
Raichle Molitar USA
RailRiders
Salomon
Seirus
Shaklee
Smart Wool
Smith Sport Optics
Sports Heat
Swiss Army Knives
Thor-Lo, Inc.
Ugg Boots
Vuarnet
Wild Country
Wrangler
YubaShoes

Resources

BOOKS

Da Silva, Rachel. *Leading Out: Women Climbers Reaching for the Top.* Seattle: Seal Press, 1992.

Evans, Laura. *The Climb of My Life.* New York: Harper Collins, 1996.

Gould, Jean. *Season of Adventure.* Seattle: Seal Press, 1996.

Graydon, Don. *Mountaineering: The Freedom of the Hills*, Fifth Edition. Seattle: The Mountaineers Books, 1992.

Secor, R. J. *Aconcagua, A Climbing Guide.* Seattle: The Mountaineers Books, 1994.

Whittaker, Lou with Andrea Gabbard. *Lou Whittaker, Memoirs of a Mountain Guide.* Seattle: The Mountaineers Books, 1994.

ORGANIZATIONS

THE BREAST CANCER FUND
Andrea Martin, Founder & Executive Director
282 Second St., Third Floor
San Francisco, CA 94105
800/487-0492; 415/543-2979 (fax)

THE EXPEDITION INSPIRATION FUND FOR BREAST CANCER RESEARCH
Laura Evans, Founder & Executive Director
P.O. Box 4289
Ketchum, ID 83340
208/726-6456; 208/726-2040 (fax)

ADVENTURE TRAVEL OUTFITTER
Peter and Erika Whittaker
Summits Adventure Travel
51902 Wanda Road
Eatonville, WA 98328
360/569-2992; 360/569-2993 (fax)

CLIMBING SCHOOL, GUIDE SERVICE
Lou Whittaker
Rainier Mountaineering, Inc.
Paradise, WA 98398
253/627-6242; 253/627-1280 (fax)

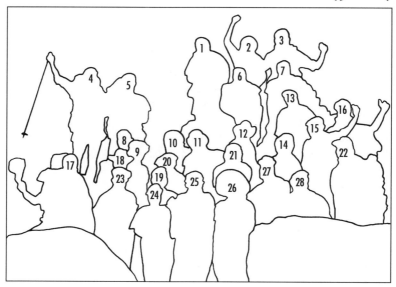

*The women and men of Expedition Inspiration after the victorious climb of
Aconcagua: 1. Dr. Bud Alpert; 2. Laura Evans; 3. Peter Whittaker; 4. Nancy
Knoble; 5. Mike "Ole" Olson; 6. Vicki Boriack; 7. Claudia Berryman-
Shafer; 8. Kurt Wedburg; 9. Jeff Martin; 10. Annette Porter; 11. Andrea
Gabbard; 12. Ashley Sumner-Cox; 13. Eleanor Davis; 14. Claudia Crosetti;
15. Nancy Johnson; 16. Paul Delorey; 17. Nancy Hudson; 18. Mary Yeo;
19. Roberta Fama; 20. Kim O'Meara Anderson; 21. Heather MacDonald;
22. Sue Anne Foster; 23. Dr. Kathleen Grant; 24. Andrea Martin; 25. Patty
Duke; 26. Sara Hildebrand; 27. Roger Evans; 28. Dr. Ron Dorn.
(Not shown: Mark "Tuck" Tucker, Erika Whittaker, Jen Wedburg, Larry and
Sue Luther, Saskia Thiadens, Ned Randolf, Catie Casson, John Hanron,
James Kay, Steve Marts, Jeannie Morris, Bill Arnold, Byron Smith.)*

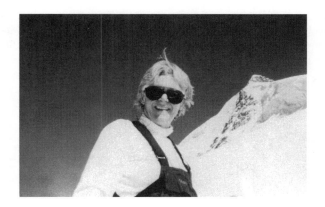

Andrea Gabbard is the co-author of the best-selling *Lou Whittaker: Memoirs of a Mountain Guide* (The Mountaineers Books, 1994) and the author of *Da-Bull: Life Over the Edge* (North Atlantic Books, 1990). A contributing editor for *Shape* and *Outdoor Retailer,* she has published hundreds of articles on outdoor subjects ranging from mountaineering to river running. She lives in the foothills of the Sierra Nevada mountains.

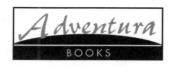

ADVENTURA BOOKS is a popular series from Seal Press that celebrates the achievements and experiences of women adventurers, athletes, travelers and naturalists. Browse the list below—and discover the spirit of adventure through the female gaze.

CANYON SOLITUDE: *A Woman's Solo River Journey Through Grand Canyon,* by Patricia C. McCairen. $14.95, 1-58005-007-7.

ANOTHER WILDERNESS: *Notes from the New Outdoorswoman,* edited by Susan Fox Rogers. $16.00, 1-878067-30-3.

SOLO: *On Her Own Adventure,* edited by Susan Fox Rogers. $12.95, 1-878067-74-5.

SEASON OF ADVENTURE: *Traveling Tales and Outdoor Journeys of Women Over 50,* edited by Jean Gould. $15.95, 1-878067-81-8.

UNCOMMON WATERS: *Women Write About Fishing,* edited by Holly Morris. $16.95, 1-878067-76-1.

A DIFFERENT ANGLE: *Fly Fishing Stories by Women,* edited by Holly Morris. $22.95, cloth, 1-878067-63-X.

FEMME D'ADVENTURE: *Travel Tales from Inner Montana to Outer Mongolia,* by Jessica Maxwell. $14.00, 1-878067-98-2.

LEADING OUT: *Women Climbers Reaching for the Top,* edited by Rachel da Silva. $16.95, 1-878067-20-6.

RIVERS RUNNING FREE: *A Century of Women's Canoeing Adventures,* edited by Judith Niemi and Barbara Wieser. $16.95, 1-878067-90-7.

WATER'S EDGE: *Women Who Push the Limits in Rowing, Kayaking and Canoeing* by Linda Lewis. $14.95, 1-878067-18-4.

ALL THE POWERFUL INVISIBLE THINGS: *A Sportswoman's Notebook,* by Gretchen Legler. $12.95, paper, 1-878067-69-9.

THE CURVE OF TIME: *The Classic Memoir of a Woman and her Children who Explored the Coastal Waters of the Pacific Northwest,* by M. Wylie Blanchet. $14.95, 1-878067-27-3.

GIFTS OF THE WILD: *A Woman's Book of Adventure,* from the editors of Adventura Books. $16.95, 1-58005-006-9.

If you are unable to obtain a Seal Press title from a bookstore, or would like a free catalog of our books, please order from us directly by calling 1-800-754-0271. Visit our website at <www.sealpress.com>.